The Morphology of Human Blood Cells

L. W. Diggs, MD; Dorothy Sturm; and Ann Bell, MS
University of Tennessee Center for Health Sciences
Department of Medicine, Division of Hematology
and Regional Medical Center
Memphis, Tennessee

FIFTH EDITION

ABBOTT LABORATORIES
Abbott Park, IL 60064

CONTENTS

PREFACE

This atlas, which portrays the morphologic characteristics of normal and pathologic cells in smears of blood and bone marrow, is published mainly for the use of medical students, student medical technologists, veterinary students, and other health-science students who are learning to identify the various types of hemic cells. This monograph also is an aid for teachers of morphologic hematology and for technologists and technicians who are responsible for the examination of smears by manual or automated methods and for the reporting of differential counts. A knowledge of morphology is also useful for residents in clinical and anatomic pathology, pediatrics, and medicine.

Major emphasis is placed on the anatomical characteristics of individual cells in the various stages of their maturation as revealed by light microscopy, employing an oil-immersion objective. Unless otherwise stated, the cells that are described and visually depicted by the artist, Dorothy Sturm, are those present in thin, air-exposed, dried smears or imprints that have been stained by a combination (Wright or equivalent stain) of the blue dye (methylene blue) and the red dye (eosin).

The procedure was to select an ideally prepared stained smear of fresh blood or aspirate of bone marrow without admixture with an anticoagulant and without fixation except by air drying and by methyl alcohol in the stain—and then to locate a typical cell in the thin portion of a smear. Dorothy Sturm, a skilled artist as well as a biologically trained scientist, painted the various colors and structures of the cells as she viewed them. Water colors were employed for the color plates.

It is impossible to portray by means of a relatively few cells all the infinite variations of nuclear and cytoplasmic structures of normal and pathologic cells. The authors have attempted to portray cells that are representative. Once selected, the cell was painted as that individual cell appeared. Unless otherwise specified, all cells are reproduced at a magnification of approximately × 1,800.

The microscopic examination of the cells of the blood and blood-forming organs is an extension of the history and physical examination. The identification and enumeration of cells in stained smears is of value as a screening procedure to detect normality as well as an aid in the diagnosis and differential diagnosis of various diseases, the establishment of prognosis, the indications for treatment, and the response to therapy—and as a safeguard against drug toxicity.

The development of new instruments and new technologies such as electron, stereoscan, and fluorescent microscopy and the employment of cytochemical, enzymatic, radioisotopic, centrifugal, serologic, electrophoretic, and other procedures have expanded our knowledge and understanding of normal and pathophysiologic mechanisms and the interpretation of morphologic characteristics as revealed by optical microscopy. These new, ingenious, important, and welcomed techniques are supplements to—not replacements of—the simple, time-honored, and relatively inexpensive microscopic procedures.

The reader is referred to textbooks of hematology for a discussion of etiologic factors, the clinical and anatomical manifestations, and the treatment of various diseases of blood and blood-forming organs. The reader is also referred to other sources for information about techniques, cell kinetics, pathophysiology, and lists of diseases characterized by an increase or decrease in the total leukocyte count and in the relative and absolute numbers of nucleated cells of different types.

Appreciation is expressed to numerous individuals who assisted in various ways in the preparation of this atlas. These include Mrs. Jane Tyler and other technologists in the special hematology laboratory at Baptist Memorial Hospital; Mrs. Lew Bailey and Mrs. Linda Mason, medical technologists at the Regional Medical Center; Mrs. Sara Cobb at St. Jude Children's Research Hospital—and from the University of Tennessee Center for the Health Sciences, Division of Hematology, Miss Helen Goodman, a hematology technologist; Miss Jeanie Peeples, research technician; and Drs. Luther Burkett, Marion Dugdale, Henry Herrod, Alfred Kraus, Alvin Mauer, Charles Neely, Gerald Plitman, and J.D. Upshaw. The authors wish to thank Mrs. Beatrice Diggs for library work, editing, and typing; Mr. Thomas Craig, from Abbott Laboratories professional relations, for his cooperation and understanding in the technical phases of the editing and printing; and Abbott Laboratories for publishing this atlas as a service to the medical profession.

L. W. Diggs, MD

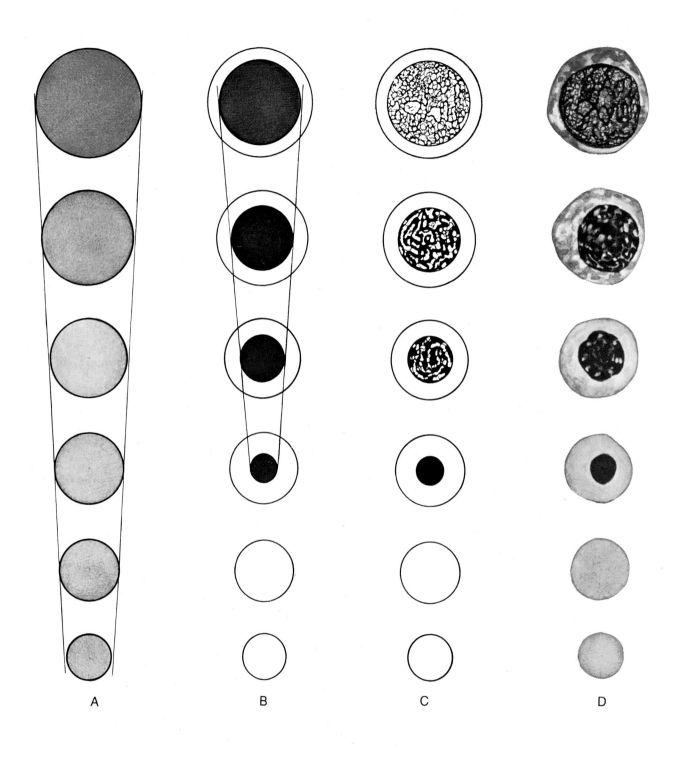

PLATE 1—MATURATION SEQUENCE

A Cell size and cytoplasm color
B Nuclear size and color
C Nuclear chromatin structure
D Composite (Top to bottom: Rubriblast,
   prorubricyte, rubricyte, metarubricyte, diffusely
   basophilic erythrocyte, erythrocyte)

CELL MORPHOLOGY – GENERAL

ALL BLOOD CELLS originate from undifferentiated mesenchymal cells (Table 1, Fig 20). From these stem cells, clones of cells differentiate and ultimately appear in the circulating blood as red cells, platelets, and various types of white cells. The earliest cells of each cell line have similar morphologic characteristics and cannot be differentiated by appearance alone. They are given specific names such as "myeloblast," "lymphoblast," or "rubriblast" depending on the tissue in which they are found, the cells with which they are associated, and the definitive cell that they are destined to produce. As the embryonic cells change from their primitive forms to mature cell types, they undergo changes in nuclear and cytoplasmic characteristics common to all cells. These changes are detailed in Plate 1.

Maturation sequence. Immature cells as a class are large and become progressively smaller as they mature (Plate 1A). The nuclei of young cells of the maturation sequence are large and relatively large in relation to the cytoplasm. As the cells age, the absolute and relative size of the nucleus decreases (Plate 1B). In cells of the erythrocytic series, the small and degenerated nuclei in the older cells are extruded.

The cytoplasm of a primitive cell is predominantly blue and contains large amounts of ribonucleic acid (RNA), which has an affinity for the basic or blue dye (methylene blue). As the cytoplasmic structures and secretory products are manufactured, the color of the cytoplasm becomes more red and less blue (Plate 1A). The nuclear chromatin strands of immature cells contain deoxyribonucleic acid (DNA), which has an affinity for the acidophilic (eosinophilic) red dye. As the nucleus ages, it stains more intensely, and the color changes from purplish-red to dark blue (Plate 1B).

The most reliable criterion of the age of a given cell and its position in the maturation sequence is the structure of the nuclear chromatin. In the most-primitive cells, the nuclear chromatin strands are distinctly visible. No part of the chromatin is darker or more compact than other portions. In some cells, the pattern is linear, whereas in others, the superimposed, tortuous and twisted chromatin threads appear as red granules or short rods. If injured in the process

of aspiration or spreading on a slide, the delicate and lacelike chromatin strands become thick and ropy but remain intact and distinct. When the nucleus degenerates, the bonds of the helical structure of the elongated DNA molecules are broken, and the chromatin strands widen and become more coarse and clumped. In the terminal degenerative and senile stages, the nucleus is small, round, dark, and structureless (Plate 1C).

One of the signs of immaturity in blood cells is the presence of nucleoli in the nucleus. These small islands of cytoplasmic material, manufactured within the nucleus, are signs of metabolic activity and growth. Nucleoli are best seen in very-thin smears and may be indistinct and obscured in thick or darkly stained smears. Nucleoli vary in number, shape, and size, but usually there are one to four nucleoli, round or oval in shape, with diameters in the 2 to 4 μm range. They have a fairly homogeneous structure and a color similar to that of the cytoplasm. In methylene blue and eosin stains, the color is predominantly blue. Nucleoli are not bounded by membranes, but the expanding intranuclear masses tend to compress the surrounding chromatin strands to give the appearance of a dark boundary (Plate 1D).

The combined changes in size and color of the cytoplasm and the size, color, and structure of the nucleus are visualized in Plate 1D.

The cytoplasmic shape of cells is influenced by the mechanical trauma to which the cells are subjected, the pressure of surrounding cells, and their ameboid activity. Primitive cells tend to be fixed by their cytoplasmic extensions in the ground substance. When torn away from their attachments, as in the process of bone marrow aspiration, the margins are disrupted, and the edges have a frayed and jagged appearance. Mature and free cells in the circulating blood usually have smooth margins. Cells of the monocytic-macrophage system are slowly motile cells that tend to adhere to glass and plastic surfaces. They continue to spread out during the drying process. These cells often reveal blunt cytoplasmic extensions (pseudopods) seldom seen in other cells. Granulocytes and lymphocytes are actively motile cells that do not stick readily to the surfaces of slides. These cells tend to round up and to become spherical when exposed to the air and as they slowly dry in the thicker portions of smears.

Table 1 – Blood Cells					
HEMATOPOIETIC TISSUES					
				CIRCULATING BLOOD	
		E. Myelocyte			Eosinophil
Myeloblast	Promyelocyte	N. Myelocyte	N. Metamyelocyte	Neutrophil Band	Neutrophil Segmented
		B. Myelocyte			Basophil
Monoblast	Promonocyte				Monocyte
Megakaryoblast	Promegakaryocyte	Megakaryocyte	Metamegakaryocyte		Thrombocyte
Rubriblast	Prorubricyte	Rubricyte	Metarubricyte	Diffusely Basophilic Erythrocyte	Erythrocyte
Lymphoblast	Prolymphocyte				Lymphocyte
Plasmoblast	Proplasmocyte			Plasmocyte	

Stem Cell

Tissue cells and early cells which move slowly have round, oval, or slightly indented nuclei. Actively motile and mature cells, such as monocytes and granulocytes, have indented, kidney-shaped, lobulated, or segmented nuclei. The nuclei of mature lymphocytes are usually round, but they may be slightly indented. The nuclei of red cells and plasma cells in all stages of maturation are round.

Immature cells that are metabolically active reveal in their cytoplasm a relatively light zone adjacent to the nucleus. This area, known as the Golgi area, contains a smooth endoplasmic reticulum and centrioles. In this juxtanuclear area, colorless (achromatic) mitochondria tend to aggregate. The light zone near the nucleus is best exemplified in plasmocytes but is visible in immature blood cells of all types.

Granules are not present in stem cells. In the series of cells that characteristically develop granules, the primary granules are dark and predominantly blue. The specific and secondary granules that later develop in the more-mature cells stain less intensely and are more red and less blue, as exemplified by eosinophils and neutrophils (Plate 3). Manufactured products within cells, such as globulin in plasmocytes or hemoglobin in red cells, are indicative of maturation.

Phagocytosis of particulate matter is a manifestation of functional activity characteristic of differentiated cells, but the absence of phagocytosis in a given cell at a given time has no value in determining the maturity of a cell.

The cytoplasmic, granular, and nuclear characteristics are usually well-synchronized in normal cells, but in pathological conditions, the maturation sequences of the various cell structures may be out of step with each other. This is the case,

for example, in the nucleated red cells of pernicious anemia which may have advanced hemoglobin synthesis and immature nuclear characteristics, or in the cells of iron-deficiency anemia, in which the hemoglobin is inadequately formed in cells with pyknotic nuclei.

Reproductive sequence. In addition to the changes in cell morphology that are manifestations of differentiation and maturation, there are morphologic changes that are manifestations of reproduction and multiplication. A few primitive cells in hematopoietic tissues remain undifferentiated and undergo mitotic division that likewise produces undifferentiated cells. Other cells, after the first mitosis, differentiate to a degree before they divide again. When these slightly more-mature cells undergo mitosis, the daughter cells maintain the cytoplasmic characteristics of the parent cells from which they derive. The majority of cells enter the mitotic cycle in the intermediate stages of maturation, as for example, in the promyelocyte or myelocyte stages of the granulocytes or the prorubricyte or rubricyte stages of the nucleated red cells. After one or several mitotic cycles, the nucleus degenerates and loses its ability to divide.

After the mitotic division of the nucleus, the cleavage of the cytoplasm, and the formation of two cells from the parent cell, the nuclear membrane re-forms around the chromosomes. The cell and its nucleus progressively enlarge. Nucleoli appear in the nucleus. During the last few hours of the division cycle, the nuclear membrane and the nucleoli disappear, and the chromatin condenses into dark, compact masses. Each chromatin thread divides, spindles extend outward from the

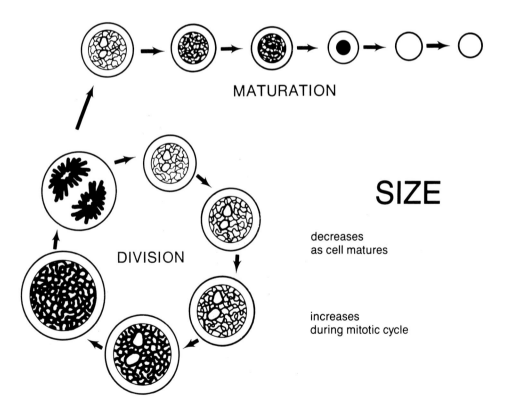

MATURATION

SIZE

decreases
as cell matures

DIVISION

increases
during mitotic cycle

Fig 1—Cell size.

centrosomes, and the chromosomes migrate to the opposite poles. Lines of cleavage appear in the cytoplasm, and two new cells are formed. At the time of mitosis, the cytoplasm, like the nucleus, is in a state of unrest and assumes a granular or bubbly appearance.

The volume of any given nucleated cell that is capable of replication at any given time is dependent on the quantity of DNA in the nucleus and the quantity of RNA and constituents in the cytoplasm. Each cell, in preparation for mitosis, approximately doubles its component of genetic material and cytoplasmic organelles before that cell divides. During the early growth (G_1) phase, the cell is appreciably smaller than that same cell will be a few hours later. During DNA synthesis (S_1) and the later growth (G_2) interval, there is a progressive increase in volume. Frequency-distribution curves of cell diameters in smears of normal, as well as pathologic, cells reveal bell-shaped curves. Between the largest and smallest cells, there are intermediate diameters. Cells that have adequate nutrition and long periods of growth between divisions are larger than are cells with inadequate nutrition, inability to utilize nutrient factors, or shortened mitotic cycles.

Mitotic figures are not demonstrable in smears of peripheral blood of individuals who are in good health. Mitotic figures in bone marrow smears of normal individuals are difficult to find. The presence of more than one cell in mitosis per 1,000 nucleated marrow cells is an indication of abnormal proliferative activity.

The cytoplasmic shape of cells throughout interphase is variable. Cells observed during the time of mitosis often have very-irregular shapes and blunt and frayed cytoplasmic protrusions caused by the violence of cytoplasmic movement during the act of tearing apart and separating.

The nuclei of cells during interphase are round. During prophase and in the later stages of mitosis (metaphase, anaphase, and telophase), the nuclear shape is irregular.

The color of the cytoplasm of undifferentiated and blast cells participating in the division cycle is blue, but in the more differentiated cells, such as hemoglobin-containing nucleated red cells or eosinophils undergoing mitosis, the color of the cytoplasm and the structures within the cytoplasm are dependent on the stage of development of the individual cell at the time it entered the reproductive cycle. Whether cells become more differentiated while they are in the premitotic phase is a moot point.

The nuclei of cells may undergo one or more mitotic divisions without the corresponding division of the cytoplasm, producing giant cells with multiple nuclei as exemplified by megakaryocytes and by double nuclei in plasmocytes and in nucleated red cells. In other cells, the chromosomes may replicate without disruption of the nuclear membrane and without division of the nucleus (endomitosis). Other abnormalities of nuclear division include: nuclei with too few or too many chromosomes; multiple nuclei within a single cell which differ in size, color, and structure; uneven number of nuclei; and clefts or cleavage lines.

Nomenclature. Nucleated cells which are morphologically undifferentiated (anaplastic) and that cannot, by associ-

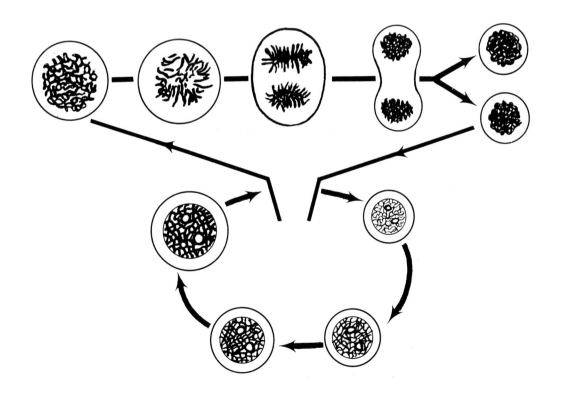

Fig 2—Mitotic cycle.

ation with other cells, be identified as blast cells of any given cell line are tallied and reported as "stem cells" (Table 1).

Each clone of definitive cells is given a family name. The suffix "blast" is reserved for the least-differentiated cells of each specific cell line. The suffix "cyte" is employed for all of the more-mature cells. The prefix "pro" is used for the second cell in the maturation sequence. Cells characterized by four maturation stages—such as myelocytic, rubricytic,

and megakaryocytic series—are given the prefix "meta" for the fourth cell (Table 4).

The most-frequently employed synonyms for nucleated red cells in their various maturation stages are given in Table 5.

The terms "reticulum cell," "reticuloendothelial cell," and "histiocyte" are purposely avoided because there is lack of agreement concerning the morphologic characteristics of blood cells designated by these names.

Table 2—Bone Marrow Cells: Normal Adult Values	
Stem cell	0-0.01%
Myeloblast	0-1
Promyelocyte	1-5
N. Myelocyte	2-10
N. Metamyelocyte	5-15
N. Band	10-40
N. Segmented	10-30
Eosinophil	0-3
Basophil	0-1
Lymphocyte	5-15
Plasmocyte	0-1
Monocyte	0-2
Other cells	0-1
Megakaryocyte	0.1-0.5
Rubriblast	0-1
Prorubricyte	1-4
Rubricyte	10-20
Metarubricyte	5-10
WBC:Nucleated RBC Ratio 4:1	

Table 3—Peripheral Blood Cells: Normal Adult Values		
	Percent	Per mm³
N. Band	1-5	50-500
N. Segmented	50-70	2,500-7,000
Eosinophil	1-3	50-300
Basophil	0-1	0-100
Lymphocyte	20-40	1,000-4,000
Monocyte	1-6	50-600

Table 4—Nomenclature							
PREFIX	SUFFIX	MYELOCYTIC SERIES	MONOCYTIC SERIES	MEGAKARYOCYTIC SERIES	ERYTHROCYTIC (RUBRICYTIC) SERIES	LYMPHOCYTIC SERIES	PLASMOCYTIC SERIES
	___blast	myeloblast	monoblast	megakaryoblast	rubriblast	lymphoblast	plasmoblast
pro___	___cyte	promyelocyte	promonocyte	promegakaryocyte	prorubricyte	prolymphocyte	proplasmocyte
	___cyte	myelocyte	monocyte	megakaryocyte	rubricyte	lymphocyte	plasmocyte
meta___	___cyte	metamyelocyte	_____	metamegakaryocyte	metarubricyte	_____	_____

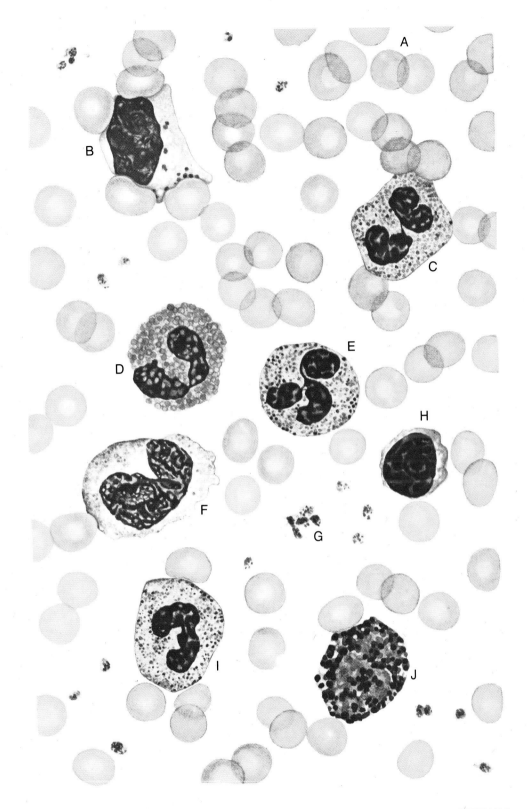

PLATE 2—CELL TYPES FOUND IN SMEARS OF PERIPHERAL BLOOD FROM NORMAL INDIVIDUALS

A Erythrocytes
B Large lymphocyte with purplish-red (azurophilic) granules
   and deeply indented by adjacent erythrocytes
C Neutrophilic segmented
D Eosinophil
E Neutrophilic segmented

F Monocyte with gray-blue cytoplasm, coarse
   linear chromatin, and blunt pseudopods
G Thrombocytes
H Lymphocyte
I Neutrophilic band
J Basophil

*The arrangement is arbitrary, and the number of leukocytes in relation to erythrocytes and
thrombocytes is greater than would occur in an actual microscopic field.*

5

II LEUKOCYTES, ERYTHROCYTES, THROMBOCYTES
Neutrophilic Leukocytes

Granular leukocytes (granulocytes) develop in the bone marrow from undifferentiated stem cells (Fig 20) and from precursor cells called myeloblasts. Maturation of the myelocytic series of cells is characterized by the development of dark and blue-staining primary granules which are later replaced by secondary granules that differ in their affinity for various dyes. Cells that have granules with an affinity for blue or basic dye are called basophils; those that are stained reddish-orange with the acid dye, eosin, are called eosinophils; and the cells with granules that do not stain intensely with either dye are called neutrophils. As the cells acquire mobility, the nuclei of the neutrophilic, eosinophilic, and basophilic systems of granular cells undergo progressive changes from round to multilobular forms designated respectively as myelocytes, metamyelocytes, band, and segmented forms (Plate 3).

Myeloblast. This cell varies in diameter from 15 to 20 μm. There is a moderate amount of bluish nongranular cytoplasm, which stains unevenly and is lighter next to the nucleus than at the periphery. Cytoplasmic tags are often demonstrable. The nucleus is round and stains predominantly red. The interlaced chromatin strands are delicate, well defined, and evenly stained. Two or more nucleoli are usually demonstrable (Plate 3).

Promyelocyte (Progranulocyte). A cell ceases to be a myeloblast and becomes a promyelocyte when it develops distinct granules (Plate 3). The earliest granules are dark-blue or reddish-blue. Most of the granules are round, but some may be elongated, curved, and irregular in shape. Granules may be visible above and below the relatively lightly stained and purple-red nucleus.

The nucleus is round or oval and relatively large in relation to the cytoplasm (Plate 3). The chromatin structure is slightly coarser, and the strands of chromatin are bluer and not as red as in the myeloblast. Nucleoli may be visible but are usually indistinct. The cytoplasm is blue with a relatively light zone adjacent to the nucleus. The cytoplasmic margins are smooth, and the cell does not indent nor is it compressed by neighboring cells. Since some early granulocytes are still capable of reproduction, the size may be quite variable, depending on the stage of a given cell in the mitotic cycle.

A promyelocyte becomes a myelocyte when the granules differentiate to such a degree that one can identify the granules as basophilic, eosinophilic, or neutrophilic.

Neutrophilic myelocyte. The first sign of neutrophilic differentiation or "dawn of neutrophilia" is the development of a small, relatively light island of ill-defined reddish granules adjacent to the nucleus (Plate 3, Plate 6). In older myelocytes, the dark granules become less prominent, and the neutrophilic granules predominate. Neutrophilic myelocytes are usually smaller than progranulocytes and have relatively larger amounts of cytoplasm. The nuclei are round, oval, or flattened on one side. The chromatin strands are unevenly stained and thickened. Nucleoli are indistinct.

Neutrophilic metamyelocyte (Juvenile). A neutrophilic metamyelocyte has a slightly indented nucleus and small, pinkish-blue granules. As a class, these cells are slightly smaller than myelocytes and have relatively smaller nuclei and less-well-defined chromatin structures (Plate 3, Plate 6). Neutrophilic metamyelocytes are rarely seen in normal peripheral blood but are often found in conditions in which there is myelocytic hyperplasia.

Neutrophilic band (N. nonsegmented, N. nonfilamented, N. staff or stab). As the neutrophilic metamyelocyte matures, the nuclear indentation becomes more marked until a stage is reached in which the indentation is greater than half the width of the hypothetical round nucleus. The opposite edges of the nucleus become approximately parallel for an appreciable distance giving a horseshoe appearance (Fig. 3). Neutrophilic bands are slightly smaller than metamyelocytes. The nucleus shows degenerative changes, and there is usually a dark pyknotic mass at each pole where the lobe is destined to be. The granules of band neutrophils are small and evenly distributed and stain various shades of pink and blue (Plate 3).

Neutrophilic band forms constitute from 1% to 5% of the leukocytes in the peripheral blood of healthy individuals. An increase in nonfilamented forms and other immature neutrophils is known as a "shift to the left" and is an indication of an abnormal response.

Neutrophilic segmented (N. filamented, N. polymorphonuclear, PMN, polymorphonuclear neutrophilic granulocyte). This cell differs from the neutrophilic band in that the nucleus is now separated into definite lobes with a very-narrow filament or strand connecting the lobes. The mature neutrophil is approximately twice the size of an erythrocyte. The cytoplasm in an ideal stain is light pink and the small, numerous, and evenly distributed granules have a light-pink to bluish-purple color (Plate 2, Plate 3).

Segmented neutrophils in the peripheral blood of older children and adults range from 50% to 70% with an average of 60%. On the average, 5% of the neutrophils have one lobe, 35% two lobes, 41% three lobes, 17% four lobes, and 2% five or more lobes. In pernicious anemia and related B_{12} and folic-acid deficiencies, there is an increase in hyperlobulated (six or more lobes) neutrophils (Plate 27, Plate 31).

The transition between the various stages of granulocytes is gradual. Many cells are borderline and difficult to distinguish from each other. The major difficulty is that of differentiating between band and segmenting forms and deciding whether the margins of the isthmus between two lobes are parallel and whether the connecting link is wide enough to be interpreted as a "band" or narrow enough to be identified as a "filament." A "band" is defined as a connecting strip or isthmus with parallel sides and wide enough to reveal two distinct margins with nuclear chromatin material visible between the margins. A "filament" is defined as a threadlike connection between two lobes so narrow that there is no visible chromatin between the two sides. In its most characteristic form, the shape of a "band" (nonsegmented, nonfilamented) nucleus is that of a bent stick, a horseshoe, or a curved link of sausage. Lobes of nuclei often touch or are superimposed so it is impossible to see connecting links. If the margin of a given lobe can be traced as a definite and continuing line from one side across the isthmus to the other side, it is assumed that a filament is present even though it is not visible (Fig 4). In differentiating between segmented (filamented) and band (nonsegmented, nonfilamented) nuclei, do not restrict evaluation to any single morphological characteristic but combine features including parallel sides and width of the connecting link, visibility of chromatin at the

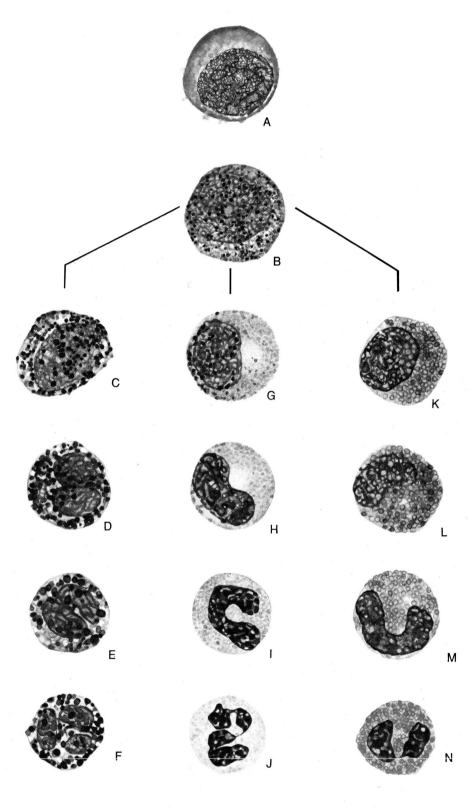

PLATE 3—MYELOCYTIC (GRANULOCYTIC) SYSTEM

A Myeloblast
B Promyelocyte (progranulocyte)

C Basophilic myelocyte	G Neutrophilic myelocyte	K Eosinophilic myelocyte
D Basophilic metamyelocyte	H Neutrophilic metamyelocyte	L Eosinophilic metamyelocyte
E Basophilic band	I Neutrophilic band	M Eosinophilic band
F Basophilic segmented	J Neutrophilic segmented	N Eosinophilic segmented

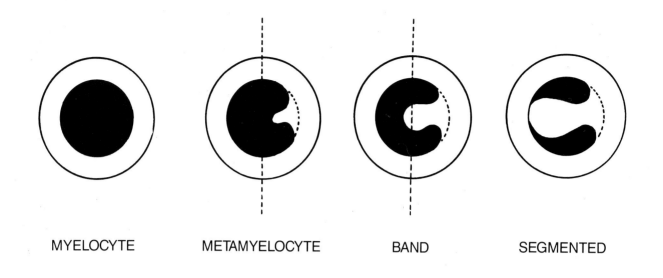

MYELOCYTE   METAMYELOCYTE   BAND   SEGMENTED

Fig 3—Terminology based on indentation of nuclei.

NONSEGMENTED

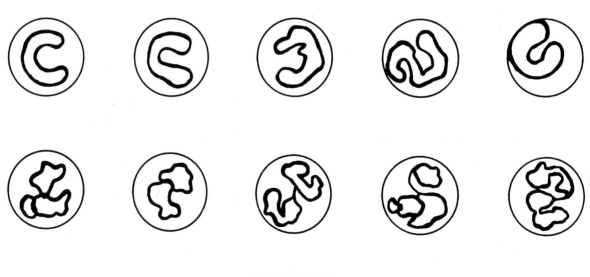

SEGMENTED

Fig 4—Neutrophil nonsegmented and segmented cells.

narrowest portion, and superimposition of lobes. In case of doubt, the rule is to place the questionable cell in the more-mature or segmented category most likely to be correct.

Morphological Abnormalities. Numerous structural abnormalities that are visible by light microscopy in the cytoplasm and nuclei of neutrophils are useful in the diagnosis and differential diagnosis of various diseases and conditions.

Hyperlobulated metamyelocytes and nonsegmented (band) neutrophils and segmented cells with five or more lobes are characteristic findings in smears of blood of patients with pernicious anemia and related B_{12}-folic acid deficiencies (Fig 5, Plate 31, Plate 27). As a rule, hyperlobulated and hypersegmented neutrophils are larger than normal cells. Hypersegmentation of giant neutrophils, as well as hyper-segmentation of cells of normal size, may be inherited characteristics.

Hypolobulation of the nuclei of neutrophils and eosinophils is a characteristic feature of the inherited and benign condition known as "Pelger-Huët anomaly." In the homozygous form, the nuclei of most of the neutrophils are round. In the heterozygous condition, the nuclei of the majority of neutrophilic leukocytes have two round lobes which are closely approximated and connected by short filaments (pince-nez form). Other nuclei are round or have dumbbell or kidney shapes (Plate 33). The nuclear chromatin and granules of hypolobulated neutrophils have normal features.

Occasionally, asynchronous Pelger-like (pseudo-Pelger) hypolobulated cells may be demonstrable in small numbers in smears of blood and bone marrow of patients with myelocytic leukemia, severe infections, or other diseases.

Prominent purplish and blue-black granules, designated as "toxic granules," often are demonstrable in the cytoplasm of neutrophils in association with severe infections and other toxic states. Toxic granules vary in size, shape, and distribution as well as in color (Plate 31). Morphologically, toxic granules resemble the primary granules of promyelocytes and early neutrophilic myelocytes. Toxic granules are manifestations of asynchronism between the maturation of nuclei and lysosomes.

Döhle bodies (Amato bodies) are inconspicuous pale sky-blue cytoplasmic inclusions. They most frequently are demonstrable in band and segmented neutrophils. Based on electron microscopic evidence, the cerulean-blue areas are residual aggregates of rough endoplasmic reticulum. Döhle bodies vary in number, distribution, and size. Some have round or oval shapes, while others appear as blue splotches with nebulous extensions. Focal areas of basophilia often are demonstrable in leukocytes that also contain "toxic granules." Döhle bodies may be demonstrable in numerous infectious diseases, as well as burns, toxemia of pregnancy, diseases due to exposure to cytotoxic chemicals, plant and animal poisons, and the hereditary May-Hegglin anomaly (Plate 36).

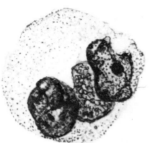
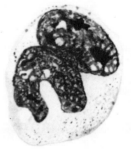
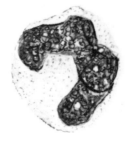
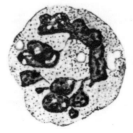

Fig 5—Hyperlobulated macroneutrophils, pernicious anemia.

The cytoplasm of neutrophils as well as other cells of patients with Alder's (Alder-Reilly) anomaly contains multiple dark-blue round or oval granules (Plate 34).

The lysosomes in the cytoplasm of granulocytes in patients with Chédiak-Higashi syndrome are grossly enlarged and vary in color from blue-black to light red and pink (Plate 35).

Auer bodies (Auer rods) are elongated narrow purplish-red structures of uncertain nature that are demonstrable in the cytoplasm of myeloblasts and monoblasts and, in rare instances, in more-mature granulocytic cells. The number in a given cell varies, but, as a rule, there is only one (Plate 40). They reveal positive reactions when peroxidase, Sudan black, and acid phosphatase stains are used. Auer rods are not demonstrable in cells of the lymphocytic, plasmocytic, erythrocytic, and megakaryocytic systems.

Spherical chromophobic areas (vacuoles) in the cytoplasm or in nuclei are manifestations of degenerative changes (Plate 31).

Lupus erythematosus is an auto-immune disease characterized by the presence of antinuclear antibodies. When aspirates of bone marrow or blood are allowed to stand outside of the body before the preparation and staining of smears, some of the nuclei in some of the leukocytes undergo lytic changes (pre-LE cells) (Plate 32). Motile neutrophils are attracted to the cells that have undergone degenerative changes. These neutrophils form clusters or rosettes around the lysed cells (Plate 32). Viable neutrophils phagocytize nuclear material, producing within the digestive vacuoles of their cytoplasm round or oval inclusions which have a fairly homogeneous structure and stain purplish-red (Plate 32). Neutrophils that contain inclusions that are reddish-purple and structureless are called LE cells. Neutrophils that have engulfed lysed nuclear masses may themselves undergo degenerative changes producing post-LE cells (Plate 32). Morphological changes of the types described above are not specific for lupus erythematosus. The final diagnosis should be based on combined clinical manifestations and other laboratory tests.

Structureless red-staining cytoplasmic inclusions of the type demonstrable in stained smears of bone marrow and body fluids in patients with lupus erythematosus are to be differentiated from linear and/or lumpy nuclei that stain dark blue and that are contained in the cytoplasm of monocytes (Plate 31). Monocytes that have ingested nonlysed nuclei are designated as "Tart cells," so named because they resemble the cells that were observed and reported in smears of bone marrow of Mr. Tart who was a patient at the Mayo Clinic.

Eosinophils

EOSINOPHILS are characterized by relatively large, spherical granules that have a particular affinity for the acid eosin stain. The earliest recognizable eosinophils have a few dark and bluish primary granules intermingled with the secondary and specific red granules. As the eosinophils pass through their various developmental stages, the bluish granules, characteristic of the progranulocyte and the early myelocyte stages, disappear (Plate 3). Because the percentage of eosinophils is usually low in bone marrow and peripheral blood smears, no useful clinical purpose is served by routinely separating the eosinophils into their various myelocyte, metamyelocyte, band, and segmented categories. On the other hand, in situations in which the eosinophils are greatly increased, an analysis of the incidence of the various stages is indicated.

The eosinophils as seen in normal peripheral blood smears are about the size of neutrophils, and usually have band or two-lobed nuclei. The granules are spherical and uniform in size. They usually are evenly distributed in the cell and fill it. Rarely do they overlie the nucleus (Plate 2, Plate 3). In good stains, the granules take a bright reddish-orange stain with brownish tints. On focusing up and down, one can bring out highlights on individual granules or reveal them as little circles. Often this spherical shape permits identification of the cell when the stain is unsatisfactory. (Eosinophils can be identified readily in moist preparations without the use of stains, because the granules are distinct, round, relatively large, and of a brownish color.) Often it is difficult to distinguish eosinophils from neutrophils when the granules of the neutrophil are prominent and stain darkly. In case of doubt, the questionable cell should be called a neutrophil. By moving to the thin part of the field (with brighter illumination)—and paying attention to the size, uniformity, and shape of the granules rather than to the color alone—one can often make distinctions that otherwise would be guesswork.

Eosinophils, like neutrophils and basophils, are derived from progenitor myeloblasts and myelocytes (Plate 3, Plate 54).

Eosinophils constitute from 1% to 3% of leukocytes in smears of peripheral blood of normal individuals. There is a relative and absolute eosinophilia in association with the invasion, migration, and encystment of animal (metazoa) parasites. Other diseases and conditions characterized by an increase in eosinophils include bronchial asthma, hay fever, Löffler's syndrome, extensive skin lesions, recovery from bacterial and other infections, chronic myelocytic and eosinophilic leukemia, and some cases of neoplastic malignancy.

Eosinopenia occurs in conditions of stress, such as shock, severe burns, and severe infections. The absence of eosinophils in blood in surgical conditions is an unfavorable omen and the presence of—or an increase in—eosinophils is a favorable sign. Eosinophils are decreased by the administration of adrenal corticosteroids.

Eosinophilic leukocytes are motile cells that are infrequently phagocytic. They leave the blood and enter tissue spaces at the sites of antigen-antibody contacts. It is thought that the histamine liberated from basophils during the initial stage of an allergic reaction serves as a chemotactic factor. Eosinophils aid in the restraint and control of inflammatory reactions. They also have cytotoxic properties against invading animal parasites.

Basophilic Leukocytes
(Basophils, Basophilic Granulocytes)

BLOOD BASOPHILS which are derived from myeloblasts and progranulocytes have round, indented, band, or segmented nuclei (Plate 2, Plate 3, Plate 54, Fig 6). Based on the shape of their nuclei, they may be classified as basophilic myelocytes, metamyelocytes, and band and segmented forms, but the cells are so few in peripheral blood and bone marrow smears that there is no clinical advantage in placing the cells in separate categories.

Blood basophils in all stages of their maturation are smaller than promyelocytes, and their size is approximately the same as that of neutrophils in the same or closely adjacent microscopic fields (Fig 6). The margins are smooth, and the shape is round or oval. Nuclei, in contrast to the darkly stained granules, are inconspicuous. The color of the nuclei is purple-red.

Basophilic granules vary in size from 0.2 to 1.0 μm. Most of the granules are round. They are numerous and unevenly distributed. The color of the granules varies from deep purplish-blue to dark purple-red. Due to intense staining, the granules stand out in sharp contrast to the light purplish color of the cytoplasm. The darkly stained granules are visible above and below the lightly stained nuclei.

The basophilic granules are water soluble. In smears, imprints, or sections of bone marrow that are exposed to moisture before being fixed or that are poorly fixed during the staining process, the granules disappear, leaving small, round, and colorless cytoplasmic areas.

Granules of the type present in basophilic leukocytes have a love or an affinity for basic dyes. When stained by a single blue dye such as toluidine blue; azure A, B, or C; or other blue and basic dyes, the granules, instead of revealing the blue color of the dye that was used, are red (metachromasia). The Wright stain contains two dyes: the red dye, eosin, and the blue dye, methylene blue. The granules of basophilic leukocytes, when stained by the Wright method, reveal varying shades of red and blue. The predominant color is blue.

The granules of basophilic leukocytes yield negative or very weak peroxidase, Sudan black, and alkaline phosphatase reactions. Some basophils react positively when periodic acid Schiff (PAS) stain is used.

Basophils differ from neutrophils and monocytes in that they are not phagocytic. The granules in basophils are membrane-bound sacks containing secretory products including heparin, histamine, and other chemicals. They are not lysosomes that contain digestive enzymes. When properly stimulated, the granules present in basophilic leukocytes eject the chemicals contained in their storage areas (exocytosis).

The number of leukocytes with basophilic granules in smears of peripheral blood or bone marrow of normal individuals is less than one per 100 nucleated cells.

The most striking relative and absolute increase in basophilic leukocytes in the peripheral blood as well as in the bone marrow occurs as a manifestation of basophilic (mast cell) leukemia. There is a relative and absolute, but less-marked, increase in the number of basophils in chronic myelocytic leukemia and in myeloblastic crisis.

Since basophils in blood and bone marrow smears are present in such small numbers, the failure to find these cells during a differential count of several hundred cells is without clinical significance.

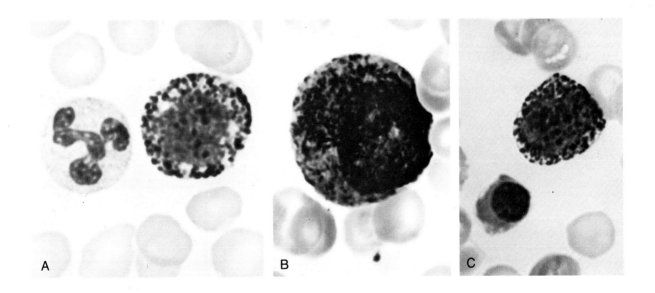

Fig 6 — A Segmented neutrophil, basophil
      B Promyelocyte
      C Nucleated red cell, basophil

Monocytes
(Large Mononuclears)

MONOCYTES are phagocytic leukocytes of the blood which, together with tissue macrophages and neutrophilic leukocytes, play a major role as a first line of defense against pathogenic organisms and nonself or foreign cells.

In smears of peripheral blood from healthy individuals, monocytes usually range from 1% to 6%. In smears of bone marrow from persons in good health, monocytes usually constitute less than 2%.

Monocytes as a class are slightly larger than neutrophils, and their diameters are three to four times those of erythrocytes in the same microscopic fields (Plate 2). Generally, there is a large amount of cytoplasm in relation to the nucleus.

The shape of monocytes is variable (Plate 4). Many are round or oval. Others reveal blunt pseudopods which are manifestations of their slow motility. These ameboid and aggressive cells continue to move while the blood film is drying and become fixed before there is time to retract their cytoplasmic extensions. The pseudopods vary in size and in number. The outer portion of the outstretched cytoplasm (ectoplasm) often has a transparent or hyaline appearance as contrasted with the granular inner cytoplasm (endoplasm).

The cytoplasm in the Wright-stained smear is dull gray-blue as contrasted with the color of the cytoplasm of neutrophils in adjacent fields which is less-intensely stained and is pink.

The granules of monocytes are usually fine, lightly stained, numerous, and evenly distributed, giving to the cells a ground-glass appearance. In other cells, there may be, in addition to the small granules, varying numbers of prominent granules. Vacuoles are often prominent in the cytoplasm. Phagocytized erythrocytes, leukocytes, nuclei, cell fragments, pigment, bacteria, and fungi may be demonstrable in digestive vacuoles.

The nucleus of the monocyte is usually round or kidney-shaped, but may be deeply indented or have two or more lobes separated by narrow filaments. One of the most distinctive and diagnostic features of the monocyte is the presence of brainlike convolutions. Another feature of the nucleus of value in identification is the tendency of the nuclear chromatin to be loose with light spaces in between the chromatin strands, giving a coarse, linear pattern in contrast to the lymphocyte with its clumped chromatin.

Monocytes are derived from stem cells in the bone marrow. As these cells grow, they are transformed into macrophages too large to pass readily through capillaries. Extremely large mononuclear phagocytes are seldom seen in blood smears but are demonstrable in body fluids other than blood. Some of the macrophages become anchored in connective tissues where they are entrapped by reticular and collagen fibers. The smaller monocytes, the larger wandering macrophages, and the semifixed or fixed phagocytes are thought to be capable of reversible transformation from one to the other.

Promonocytes and Monoblasts are not identifiable as such in bone marrow or peripheral blood smears except in conditions in which there is marked proliferation of cells of the monocytic type as in monocytic leukemia. The identification of early mononuclear cells is based on the indented and folded nuclei and the association with more mature monocytes having blunt pseudopods, vacuoles, and phagocytic particles in the cytoplasm. The cells in monocytic leukemia are called monoblasts when the nuclear chromatin

is fine and distinct, nucleoli are demonstrable, and there are no granules in the cytoplasm (Plate 41).

Monocytes vs Neutrophils vs Large Lymphocytes. Monocytes are the cells of the peripheral blood most difficult to identify and to differentiate from other cells (Plate 6). They are frequently mistaken for neutrophils, for they may have prominent granules and lobulated nuclei. The monocyte often is mistaken for a large lymphocyte, because its cytoplasm is blue, or because the granules may be indistinct, the nucleus round or only slightly indented, the linear chromatin pattern ill defined, and the distinctive blunt pseudopods and digestive vacuoles missing.

The three most characteristic features of the monocyte and the most helpful in diagnosis are the dull gray-blue color of the cytoplasm, the blunt pseudopods, and the brainlike convolutions of the nucleus.

The color of the cytoplasm must not be compared with a textbook picture or hypothetical ideal cells, but with known neutrophils in the same or adjacent fields. The cytoplasm of a neutrophil is relatively light and reddish in comparison with the cytoplasm of the monocyte which is relatively dark, more bluish, and more opaque. Neutrophils practically never have blunt pseudopods.

To distinguish monocytes from large lymphocytes, the nuclear structure, the character of the cytoplasm, and the shape of the cells are most useful. The nucleus of a lymphocyte tends to be clumped, rather than linear (Plate 6). There is a greater tendency for the nuclear chromatin to be condensed at the periphery in the lymphocyte. Brainlike convolutions are not present in the lymphocyte. Monocytes and large lymphocytes may have distinct bluish-red granules (lysosomes). In addition, the cytoplasm of the monocyte has a finely granular or ground-glass appearance, whereas the cytoplasm of the lymphocyte has a background that is nongranular.

Monocytes tend to indent and to compress adjacent cells rather than to be indented by them. Large lymphocytes, on the other hand, are often deeply indented by neighboring cells (Plate 2, Plate 5).

Morphological Abnormalities. Extremely large monocytes (macrophages) in smears of peripheral blood may be demonstrable in patients with subacute bacterial endocarditis and other chronic infectious states. These large cells, some of which may contain phagocytized particulate matter, are most likely to be found at the feather edge of smears made from blood of the ear rather than from other sites.

In its cytoplasm, a monocyte may contain intact and hemoglobin-containing red cells, red-cell fragments, and hemosiderin granules, as well as phagocytized leukocytes and leukocyte fragments.

Alveolar monophagocytes ingest and degrade pathogenic organisms. They also phagocytize particles containing inspired air and serve as a means of transportation of pollutants by ciliated epithelial cells lining the respiratory tract.

Phagocytic cells of varying size and mobility remove from the circulating blood injured and dead cells, cell fragments, microorganisms, and insoluble particles. Motile monophagocytes escaping between epithelial lining cells of the upper and lower respiratory tracts and the gastrointestinal and genitourinary organs perform a scavenger function, clearing the body of insoluble and unneeded debris.

An important function of micromonocytes as well as macromonocytes (macrophages) is to ingest and kill pathogenic organisms and to ingest and degrade noxious external agents. Monophagocytes also play a role in phagocytizing old and degenerated cells and cell fragments, malignant cells, and cells that spontaneously undergo mutations in the body.

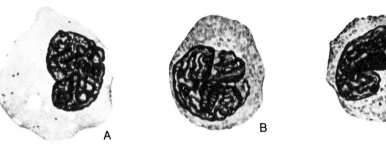

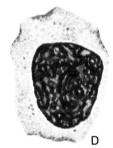 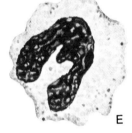 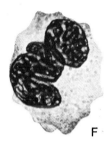

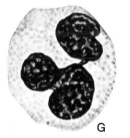 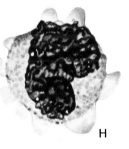 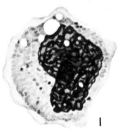

PLATE 4—MONOCYTES

A Monocyte with "ground-glass" appearance, evenly distributed fine granules, occasional azurophilic granules, and vacuoles in cytoplasm

B Monocyte with opaque cytoplasm and granules and with lobulation of nucleus and linear chromatin

C Monocyte with prominent granules and deeply indented nucleus

D Monocyte without nuclear indentations

E Monocyte with gray-blue color, band type of nucleus, linear chromatin, blunt pseudopods, and granules

F Monocyte with gray-blue color, irregular shape, and multilobulated nucleus

G Monocyte with segmented nucleus

H Monocyte with multiple blunt nongranular pseudopods, nuclear indentations, and folds

I Monocyte with vacuoles and with nongranular ectoplasm and granular endoplasm

13

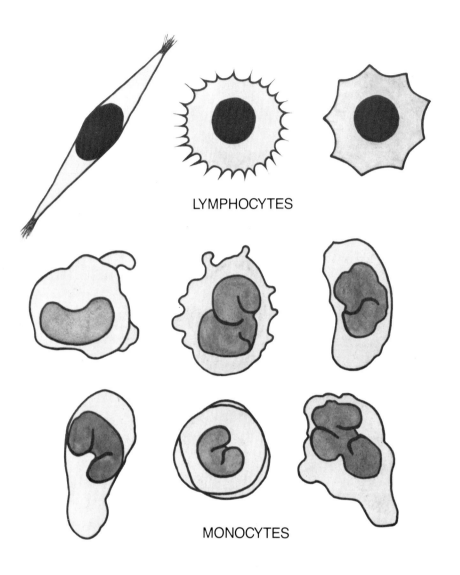

LYMPHOCYTES

MONOCYTES

Fig 7—Cell shapes.

Lymphocytes

LYMPHOCYTES are the predominant cells in the lymph and are the second most-frequently-occurring leukocytes of the blood. During the first few years of life, while children are developing immunity to infectious agents and other foreign environmental factors, lymphocytes constitute 30% to 70% of leukocytes in peripheral blood smears and 10% to 30% in bone marrow smears. In older children and adults, lymphocytes constitute from 20% to 40% of the leukocytes in peripheral blood smears and 5% to 15% of the nucleated cells in bone marrow smears. The total number of lymphocytes in the blood of individuals in good health varies from 1.5 to 4.0 x 10⁹/L.

Small Lymphocytes. The traditional and textbook descriptions of lymphocytes relate to cells in the resting or dormant stages demonstrable in smears of bone marrow, blood, or other body fluids of individuals in good health and/or those who are not exposed to antigenic stimuli. These latent cells maintain metabolic activity sufficient for survival, but they are not immunologically functional. Some of the lymphocytes that appear to be old and degenerate—because their nuclei are darkly stained, the chromatin condensed, and nucleoli invisible—have the capacity, after activation by antigens, of transforming into cells that are immunologically functional. Small lymphocytes with round nuclei and blue nongranular cytoplasm are identified and morphologically differentiated from other nucleated cells by the characteristics they lack rather than the anatomical features they reveal.

The diameters of small lymphocytes are in the 7 to 10 μm range. The nucleus in relation to the cytoplasm is large. The size of the nucleus of small lymphocytes is comparable to the diameters of normal red cells in the same microscopic fields. Small lymphocytes usually have a narrow rim of cytoplasm.

The nuclear chromatin in small lymphocytes is clumped and darkly stained. Thin sections of small lymphocytes examined by electron microscopy reveal the presence of nucleoli in some of the cells, depending on the metabolic activity of any given cell at the time of fixation. Nucleoli that may be present in older lymphocytes are not visible by light microscopy because they are obscured by dense chromatin masses. The fact that nucleoli are present in some small lymphocytes is proof of metabolic activity and the capacity of these cells for growth and replication.

Small lymphocytes usually have round shapes and smooth cytoplasmic margins (Plate 5B). Some small lymphocytes reveal a few small and pointed cytoplasmic protrusions (Plate 5G). One of the shapes seldom seen in nucleated cells other than lymphocytes is the spindle form with oval and centrally located nuclei and with tapering filaments extending outward at each end (Plate 5F). In some conditions—such as lymphocytic leukemias—in which there are numerous lymphocytes, there are multiple spindle-shaped lymphocytes with their long axes parallel, resembling schools of swimming fish.

The color of the cytoplasm is blue. The intensity of the blue color in different cells varies from light to dark. The color is evenly distributed in some cells and is uneven and splotchy in others. As a rule, the intensity of the stain is greater at the margins than in the central portions. Transmitted light deflected by the deeply stained nuclei tends to highlight the cytoplasm adjacent to the nucleus, producing a perinuclear "silver lining" or "halo" effect (Plate 5B, Plate 6F).

Lymphoblasts and Prolymphocytes. Lymphoblasts, prolymphocytes, and small lymphocytes have similar morphologic characteristics in that each has a relatively large, round or slightly indented nucleus and blue cytoplasm. The nuclei of nonfunctioning cells become progressively smaller as the cells mature (Plate 7, left column). Differentiation of cells in a maturation sequence is based principally on differences in nuclear structure. In lymphoblasts, the chromatin strands are thin, evenly stained, and reddish-purple. One or several nucleoli are demonstrable (Plate 7, Plate 39). In mature lymphocytes, the nucleus stains darkly and the chromatin is lumpy. Nucleoli in prolymphocytes are usually less distinct than in lymphoblasts, and the chromatin color and structure are intermediate. These differences are subtle. It is often a matter of opinion as to the category in which individual lymphocytic cells should be placed. In case of doubt whether a given cell is a lymphocyte, a prolymphocyte, or a lymphoblast, identify it as a lymphocyte.

Large Lymphocytes. In addition to small lymphocytes with pachychromatic nuclei and small amounts of bluish nongranular cytoplasm, there are—in smears of peripheral blood of normal individuals—a few large lymphocytes, some of which contain granules. The largest lymphocytes have diameters two to three times those of small lymphocytes in the same microscopic fields. In addition to the large and small lymphocytes, there are intermediate sizes. The number of large lymphocytes in the smears of normal peripheral blood usually ranges between 5% and 10% of the number of lymphocytes.

The diameters of nuclei of large lymphocytes, in relation to the nuclei of small lymphocytes, are significantly increased. The shape, staining characteristics, and chromatin structure are similar to those described above for small lymphocytes. Nucleoli, as a rule, are not visible by light microscopy.

The margins of large lymphocytes are often indented by erythrocytes, producing serrated, scalloped, or holly-leaf shapes (Plate 5J,K,L). Whether the marginal indentations are manifestations of the plasticity and easy compressibility of the cytoplasm or are due to the affinity of red cells and lymphocytes is not known.

The light-blue cytoplasm of some lymphocytes on casual examination is structureless, but on critical illumination and by using a superior oil-immersion system, there are fine, bluish interlacing fibrils. Areas between these fine reticular and weblike strands take a relatively light stain (Plate 5, Plate 6, Plate 7).

Some large lymphocytes contain a few unevenly distributed granules. The size of individual granules is approximately the same. The granules are spherical, have a purplish-red color, and often have a clear zone or halo around them. The granules in lymphocytes have been designated as "azurophilic," but this term is misleading because the color is predominantly red rather than blue. This is due to the fact that the blue dye stains this type of granule a red color (metachromasia). The granules in lymphocytes differ from those in neutrophilic leukocytes in that they are less numerous, are unevenly distributed, and are peroxidase- and Sudan black B-negative rather than positive. Granules in lymphocytes are acid phosphatase positive.

The role that large lymphocytes play in immunologic reactions and their relationship to small lymphocytes and to lymphoblasts is veiled in mystery. On the basis of the structure of nuclei and in the presence of well-defined granules in the cytoplasm of some of the cells, it is obvious that these cells are mature variants. It is probable that large lymphocytes, in contrast to small lymphocytes, are immunologically functional as units in bodily defense. The survival time of

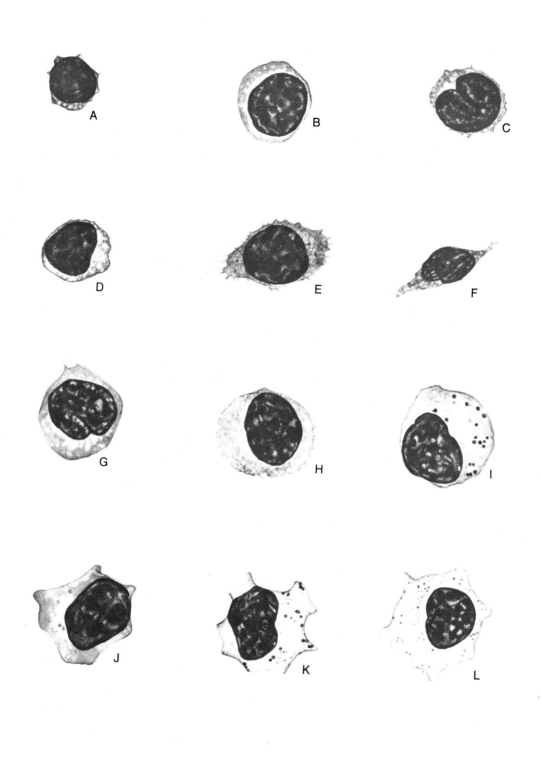

PLATE 5—LYMPHOCYTES

A Small mature lymphocyte
B Lymphocyte of intermediate size
C Lymphocyte with indented nucleus
D Lymphocyte of intermediate size
E Lymphocyte with pointed cytoplasmic projections (frayed cytoplasm); typical nucleus
F Spindle-shaped lymphocyte with indented nucleus
G Large lymphocyte with indented nucleus and pointed cytoplasmic projections

H Large lymphocyte
I Large lymphocyte with purplish-red (azurophilic) granules
J Large lymphocyte with irregular cytoplasmic contours
K Large lymphocyte with purplish-red (azurophilic) granules and with indentations caused by pressure of erythrocytes
L Large lymphocyte with purplish-red (azurophilic) granules

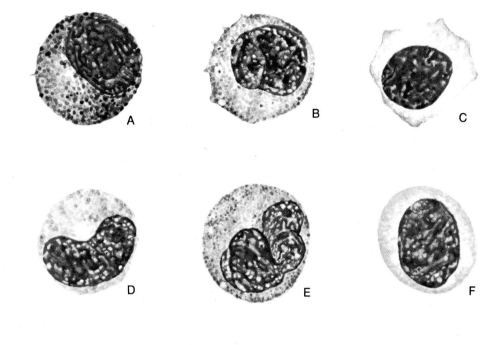

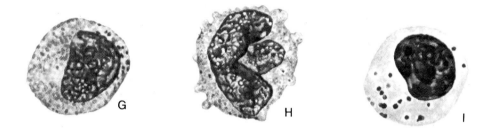

PLATE 6—COMPARATIVE MORPHOLOGY:
NEUTROPHILIC GRANULOCYTES, MONOCYTES, LYMPHOCYTES

A N. myelocyte with mixture of neutrophilic and dark reddish-purple granules
B Monocyte with nuclear fold
C Large lymphocyte with scalloped shape and absence of folds in nucleus
D N. metamyelocyte with light-pink cytoplasm color and neutrophilic granules
E Monocyte with gray-blue cytoplasm, prominent granules and multilobulated nucleus (brainlike convolutions), and linear chromatin strands

F Large lymphocyte with nongranular cytoplasm
G N. myelocyte
H Typical monocyte with lobulated nucleus, gray-blue color, and blunt pseudopods
I Large lymphocyte with purplish-red (azurophilic) granules and lumpy nuclear structure

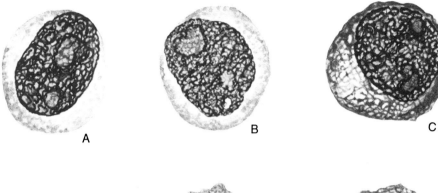

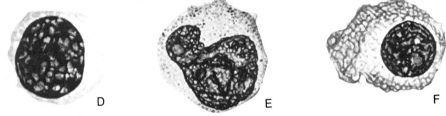

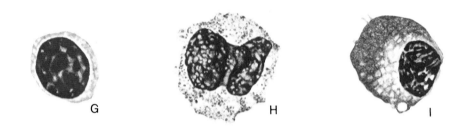

PLATE 7—LYMPHOCYTIC, MONOCYTIC, AND PLASMOCYTIC SYSTEMS

A Lymphoblast
B Monoblast
C Plasmoblast
D Prolymphocyte
E Promonocyte

F Proplasmocyte
G Lymphocyte with
  clumped chromatin
H Monocyte
I Plasmocyte

large lymphocytes is not known. Since these cells have large amounts of cytoplasm, it is unlikely that they recirculate, as do some small lymphocytes from the blood stream, into tissue spaces of lymph nodes and back again into the blood stream via lymphatic channels.

There is no useful purpose served by reporting so-called "large" and "small" lymphocytes because there are no established criteria for separation according to size. However, if there is a striking increase in large lymphocytes, with or without granules, this abnormality should be included in the laboratory report.

Activated and Reactive Lymphocytes. Some small lymphocytes have darkly stained pachychromatic nuclei and relatively small amounts of bluish nongranular cytoplasm and appear to be old by conventional morphological criteria. However, they prove not to be old when they are stimulated by appropriate antigens and are shown to be capable of rejuvenation and transformation into cells that grow, proliferate, and evolve into cells that are immunologically competent.

The size of transformed lymphocytes varies (Plate 38), but usually they are significantly larger than the small lymphocytes from which they are derived. The increase in volume in the later phases of preparation for mitosis is due to an increase in DNA in the nuclei and RNA in the cytoplasm. There also is an increase in rough endoplasmic reticulum and in the number and size of mitochondria. In some large reactive cells, granules are present. The nuclei of some of the lymphocytes that are responding to activation by antigens have leptochromatic (blastlike) nuclei and visible nucleoli.

Smears of peripheral blood and bone marrow of patients whose lymphocytes are activated by antigens may reveal large monocytoid cells (? lymphocyte, ? monocyte) with oval, indented, or lobulated nuclei; granular cytoplasm; vacuoles; and blunt pseudopods (Plate 37). Lymphocytes that respond to antigenic stimuli constitute a heterogeneous population or wide spectrum of morphologic variants (Plate 38). There is no single term that can possibly describe all types of reactive cells any more than one color can adequately describe a rainbow.

The most striking variants, and the greatest number of transformed or reactive lymphocytes, are demonstrable in the smears of peripheral blood of patients with infectious mononucleosis, a febrile lymphoproliferative disease which is usually relatively benign and self limiting. The etiologic agent is the Epstein-Barr virus (EBV). During the first few days, there may be a slight neutropenia, but by the time the patient seeks medical care, the total leukocyte count is usually slightly elevated. Small to intermediate lymphocytes usually constitute 60% or more of the leukocytes. The majority of lymphocytes have normal nuclear and cytoplasmic characteristics. There are occasional large granular lymphocytes and reactive cells of all types (Plate 37, Plate 38). The cytoplasm in some of the cells has a bubbly appearance. Vacuoles may be present. In rare instances, mitotic figures may be demonstrable.

The bizarre lymphocytic, plasmocytic, and monocytic variants; blastoid cells; and mitotic figures that may be present in association with the more-severe forms of infectious mononucleosis may simulate the cytoplasmic changes observed in patients with lymphoblastic leukemia. Morphologically similar cells may be present in both diseases. The main differences lie in the repetitious types of pathologic cells in leukemic states and the striking mixture of leukocytes of various types in infectious mononucleosis. In the blood picture in infectious mononucleosis, there are—in addition to an increase in small lymphocytes with normal morphologic characteristics—intermediate and large lymphocytes; reactive lymphocytes of all types; as well as neutrophils, monocytes, and occasional eosinophils and basophils. As a rule, there are no nucleated red cells. Thrombocytes are present in normal numbers. These signs are extremely helpful in diagnosis between benign and malignant conditions. In leukemic states, the normal bone marrow cells usually are replaced by malignant cells. The bone marrow in patients with infectious mononucleosis may reveal granulomatous areas in tissue sections, but there is no replacement of marrow cells by lymphocytes.

Viruses other than the EBV of infectious mononucleosis that are characterized by an increased proliferation of reactive lymphocytes include the cytomegalovirus and the etiologic agents of hepatitis, herpes zoster (shingles), viral pneumonia, lymphocytic choriomeningitis, mumps, rubeola, rubella, chicken pox, and smallpox. Reactive lymphocytes are demonstrable in a host of other diseases and conditions, such as auto-immune diseases, reactions to drugs and plant and animal poisons, allergic skin diseases, serum sickness, post-transfusion reactions, organ transplants, and infections due to protozoa, fungi, spirochetes, and rickettsiae. Reactive lymphocytes are demonstrable also during the recovery phase of bacterial infections.

Since malignant cells of various types are foreign to the body, it is possible to find reactive lymphocytes in association with leukemias, lymphomas, and other malignant diseases.

It is recommended that large lymphocytes with varying degrees of cytoplasmic basophilia and those with immature nuclear characteristics, abnormal shapes, and unusual cytoplasmic structures be reported on the laboratory report form as "lymphocyte variants." This term is preferable to "atypical lymphocytes," because the morphologic changes that occur in lymphocytes which respond to antigenic stimulants are typical of immunologically functional cells, although they are not typical of cells that are in the resting or dormant phase.

Eponyms such as "Türk irritation cells" and "Downey I, II, and III" should not be used. It is difficult enough for students to remember descriptive terms without having to remember the names of famous hematologists who years ago first described morphologic variants. The term, "pyroninophilic cells," is taboo unless the supravital stain, "pyronin," was actually employed and the cytoplasm revealed an affinity for the red dye. "Virocyte" is an unacceptable term because while it is true that reactive cells often are present in association with viral diseases, the same types of reactive cells also are present in nonviral diseases and conditions.

The pathologist responsible for the anatomical diagnosis and the clinician responsible for the clinical diagnosis and establishment of prognosis and treatment have the freedom to employ any interpretive changes they may choose, including terms that imply assumed trigger factors such as "activated," "stimulated," "sensitized," "irritated," or "turned on." Physicians are also justified in employing terms such as "reactive," "transformed," "transitional," and "rejuvenated." The person responsible for the report of the differential leukocyte count should not employ terms that involve etiology, response to antigenic stimuli, or function.

T and B Lymphocytes (Fig 8, Fig 9). The first cells to be identified as blood cells are large (macrocytic, megalocytic), hemoglobin-containing nucleated red cells that appear in the yolk sac along with endothelial cells of primitive blood vessels during the early weeks of embryonic life. Hematopoiesis involving erythrocytes, granulocytes, monocytes, and megakaryocytes occurs after the second month of fetal life. The hematopoietic organs that are next involved in the production of blood cells are the liver, spleen, bone marrow, thymus, and lymph nodes in that order.

Morphologically undifferentiated progenitor cells (stem cells) that proliferate in fetal hematopoietic organs, including the marrow, are transported by the blood to various anatomical sites. Some of these migrant cells lodge in the thymus, an epithelial organ of the upper gastrointestinal tract. Stem cells that come in contact with epithelial cells and grow and reproduce in the thymus have the anatomical characteristics of lymphocytes. Some of the thymus-related or thymus-dependent cells are seeded into lymph nodes, spleen, bone marrow, and other organs.

During postnatal life, all types of blood cells, including some of the lymphocytes and plasmocytes, are produced in the bone marrow. However, most of the lymphocytes and plasmocytes are derived from proliferating progenitor cells in the lymph nodes, tonsils, and thymus; and lymphoid tissues in the spleen, the mucosal areas of the intestine, and the respiratory and genitourinary tracts, as well as other extramedullary organs.

Thymus-related T lymphocytes are responsible for immunity of the cellular type (Fig 8). These cells function by establishing direct contact with undesired foreign (nonself) cells and inhibiting the growth of, or killing, alien cells. In cooperation with other cells of the immune system, T cells aid in the defense of the body against viral, fungal, and other infections; in the rejection of grafts; and in the inhibition of growth or the destruction of body cells that have undergone spontaneous and undesired mutations. T cells also provide the necessary help for B lymphocytes to differentiate into antibody-producing cells. In persons whose defense mechanisms are depressed by total-body irradiation or by cytotoxic drugs and who receive bone marrow transfusions, the T cells of the donor may predominate over those of the recipient, resulting in graft-vs-host (runt) disease. When organs are transplanted, the cytotoxic cells of the host attempt to reject the graft. T cells also participate in delayed sensitivity reactions.

The most-readily available, least-expensive, and most-frequently employed procedure for the identification of T lymphocytes is the sheep erythrocyte rosette (E-rosette) test. This test is performed by incubating a solution rich in lymphocytes with sheep erythrocytes which have an affinity for, and cluster around, T cells. Approximately 70% to 80% of the lymphocytes in the peripheral blood of normal individuals form E-rosettes.

Research has revealed that undifferentiated mesenchymal cells (stem cells) originating in various fetal hematopoietic organs migrate in the blood to the cloaca (bursa of Fabricus) of chickens where these progenitor cells come in contact with the epithelial cells of the hind gut. Cells having the morphologic characteristics of lymphocytes proliferate in, and are delivered from, the bursa into the blood. These cells are transported to, and transplanted in, lymph nodes and other lymphoid organs where they grow and multiply. Lymphocytes that have come under the influence of epithelial cells of the bursa of fowl are designated as "bursa-related" or B cells. The primary or central organ of the so-called B cells in mammals is not known.

It is justified to employ the term "bursa equivalent" when referring to B lymphocytes in man, but it is erroneous and inappropriate to identify B cells as "bone-marrow lymphocytes" because the spelling of "bone marrow" happens to start with a "B" or because the marrow is the place where some stem cells reside. Some of the stem cells that are the progenitor cells of thymus-related T cells during fetal life also originate in the bone marrow. During postnatal life, most lymphocytes of all types (T, B, and null) are produced in lymphoid areas other than the bone marrow, and relatively few are produced in lymphoid islands within marrow spaces.

Some lymphocytes of B lineage, after stimulation by an antigen, respond by transforming into cells with basophilic cytoplasm and with blastoid nuclear chromatin patterns. These plasmalike cells (proplasmocytic, plasmocytoid) develop within a few days into functioning plasma cells. These cells manufacture and secrete into the plasma various types

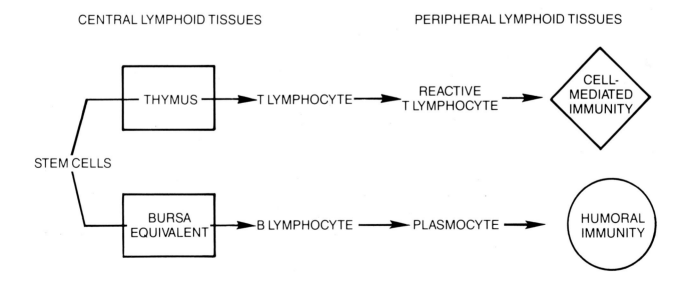

Fig 8—Lymphocytic system and immunity.

of immunoglobulins. Immunoglobulins in body fluids are designated as "humoral antibodies." The humoral immunity that is provided by plasmocytes is in contrast to "cellular immunity" provided by T lymphocytes.

B lymphocytes may be identified by the reaction that is observed after a suspension of lymphocytes is combined with fluorescein-conjugated antiserum. With this method, using fluorescent microscopy, it has been noted that 10% to 15% of the circulating lymphocytes have surface-membrane immunoglobulin and are B cells.

Additional Information. During recent years, there has been an explosive and fantastic development of new instruments and complicated, sophisticated, and expensive technical procedures to determine the functional characteristics of lymphocytes and other blood cells. Lymphocytes of the T and B cell lineage are identified and their relative numbers estimated by panels of membrane markers to detect specific antigen contained within the cytoplasm or attached to the membranes of cells. Lymphocytes that do not reveal membrane characteristics of either T or B lymphocytes are designated as "null cells."

Although opinions differ concerning the origin and the relationship of various families of blood cells and the maturation sequence of blood cells, it is generally agreed that lymphocytes and plasmocytes are closely related cells; that progenitor cells of plasma cells, as well as lymphocytes, reside in lymphoid organs; and that these cells have morphologic characteristics and immunologic functions that are different from nonlymphoid blood cells (Fig 10).

Under conditions in which there are increased demands for the proliferation of cells in hematopoietic organs, the areas occupied by fat cells in the marrow are first replaced by proliferating hemic cells. If the stimulus is great enough, production of blood cells may occur in the liver and spleen. In some cases, the proliferation also involves the creation of new marrow in the form of nodular tumorlike tissues usually located in the costovertebral areas. In malignancies involving myeloid cells, the lymph nodes—as well as nonhematopoietic organs such as the kidney, brain, skin, and other areas—are involved in the proliferative process. In lymphoid malignancies, multiple organs, including the bone marrow, are involved in the proliferative process.

In all biological systems, there are regulatory factors or forces that aid in production, growth, and development and factors that restrain and inhibit, thus making it possible to establish equilibrium and to maintain life. Thymus-related lymphocytes help B cells, plasmocytes, and phagocytic cells in fulfilling their immunological functions. Cells that assist are designated as "helpers" or "inducers." Other T cells down-regulate the activity of immune reactions and are known as "suppressors" or "inhibitors." Technical procedures with monoclonal antibodies have been developed that make it possible to determine the percentage of T cells that are helpers and those that are suppressors (the so-called H/S ratio). It has been stated that T lymphocytes that possess cytotoxic capabilities, those that provide helper activity, and those that suppress immunological reactions are different cells and that any given cell does not possess multiple capabilities.

Most leukocytes survive only a few hours or days after delivery into the circulating blood or tissues. Some lymphocytes, especially T lymphocytes, have a prolonged life expectancy and may survive months or years, retaining their reproductive capacity and ability to participate in immune reactions. It is not possible to determine the age of any given lymphocyte by its appearance in stained smears.

Lymphocytes that have a long life-expectancy migrate from the blood stream between and through the endothelial cells of capillaries and venules and through the basement membranes of blood vessels into the tissue spaces of lymph nodes. These cells later traverse the lining cells of lymph vessels. Then they are transported by efferent lymph channels into the

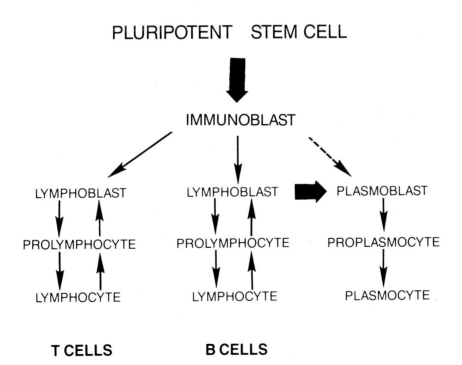

Fig 9—Lymphocytic-plasmocytic systems.

thoracic duct. The thoracic duct empties into the right innominate vein. Continual recirculation of lymphocytes from the blood into tissue spaces and back into the circulating blood favors the exposure of lymphocytes to antigens, the dissemination of antibody proteins, and the contact of effector cells with pathogenic organisms and with undesired cells. It is possible and probable that lymphocytes, in the process of passage through endothelial cells (emperipolesis) and through narrow reticular spaces, continually lose portions of their membranes and cytoplasm, thus accounting for the paucity of the cytoplasm in small lymphocytes.

Lymphocytes have the ability to pass between or through epithelial cells of the gastrointestinal tract and into the lumen of the gut. In so doing, they serve as a means of protection for the body against enteric microbial pathogens.

Lymphocytes that have been in contact with antigens and have responded by participating in immune reactions acquire the capability of retaining a memory of this immunological experience. Such lymphocytes also possess the capability of transferring "immunological memory" to successive generations of daughter cells. Descendants of previously challenged lymphocytes, when again confronted by antigens of the same type at a later date, respond more rapidly and more effectively to the later challenge than at the time of the original contact.

It is not possible on the basis of morphologic characteristics of lymphocytes to differentiate T cells, B cells, and null cells, or to determine which cells are helpers or suppressors, and which cells have the potential to evolve into killer cells or producers of immunoglobulins. The fact that the future functions of lymphocytes are not revealed by microscopic procedures in no way detracts from the valuable information that is revealed by simple, readily available, and affordable procedures.

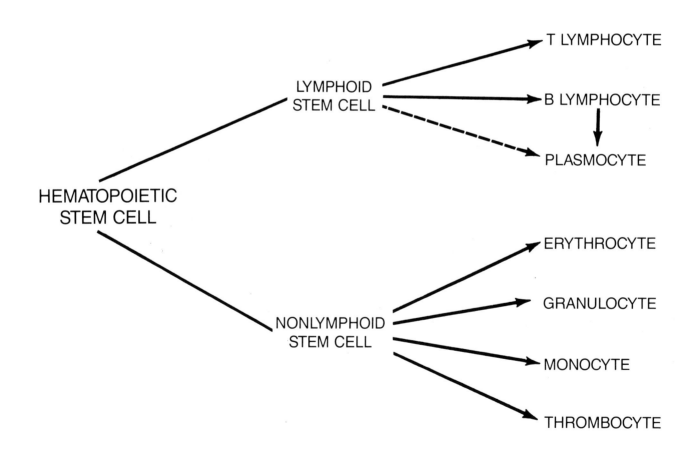

Fig 10—Lineage of lymphoid and nonlymphoid cells.

Plasmocytes
(Plasma Cells)

Leukocytes morphologically identified as lymphocytes and plasmocytes help and control each other and, in collaboration with phagocytic granulocytes and cells of the monocytic-macrophage system, are essential in the defense of the body against bacteria, viruses, spirochetes, rickettsiae, fungi, protozoa, and animal parasites. Without these cells, survival would not be possible in a hostile and competitive biological world. The combined action of defensive cells also serves as a barrier to the growth of cells foreign to the body, to malignant cells, to the destructive action of plant and animal poisons, to toxic chemicals, and to other noxious agents.

Plasmocytes constitute approximately 1% of the nucleated cells of the normal bone marrow but are not seen in the peripheral blood smears of healthy adults. They may be present in the circulating blood of young children and in the blood of patients with viral infections including exanthemas, herpes, viral hepatitis, and infectious mononucleosis. Plasmocytes are also observed in those with serum sickness, allergic states, chronic bacterial and fungal infections, toxoplasmosis, and multiple myeloma (Fig 12). In plasmocytic leukemia, in occasional auto-immune states, and in situations in which the immune system is suddenly challenged by antigenic materials, the plasmocytes may be markedly increased.

Mature plasma cells, when found in blood smears, vary in size from 15 to 25 μm. They are usually round or oval with smooth or slightly irregular margins. The cytoplasm is non-granular and stains a dark blue. In addition the cytoplasm has a brilliant translucency. This rich and velvety quality—variously described as cornflower, larkspur, or pigeon blue—is thought to be due to numerous relatively unstained mitochondria and to lightly stained or reddish secretory products that allow the light to be transmitted through the cytoplasm containing numerous dark-blue (basophilic) ribosomes. The cytoplasm adjacent to the nucleus is relatively pale (perinuclear clear zone). Fibrillar structures that take a blue stain may be demonstrable (Plate 7, right column). In many plasmocytes, there are one or several vacuoles. There is no evidence of phagocytosis of visible particles.

The nuclei of mature plasmocytes are relatively small, oval or round, and eccentric. The nuclear chromatin is coarse and lumpy.

In tissues fixed in formaldehyde or other fixatives and perhaps poorly dehydrated in the process of staining, there may be produced in the nuclei artifacts characterized by the tendency of the chromatin to clump and to adhere to the nuclear membrane, giving the vague visual impression of the spokes of a wheel. In stained blood and marrow smears, aggregates of chromatin are demonstrable in some mature cells, but "cart wheels" are figments of the imagination. The use of the phrase "cart-wheel nucleus" is a cliché copied from older textbooks of pathology, and it should be discarded.

Most plasmocytes in bone marrow are fixed or semifixed cells which are torn in the process of aspiration and appear in marrow smears with irregular spiculate margins (Plate 46). Plasmocytes in the marrow are often seen in groups clustered around large nongranular or finely granular tissue cells (Fig 11). It is thought that the contact of plasmocytes with large histiocytic cells is a manifestation of the immune response in which antigenic material, processed by macrophages, is transferred to the plasma cells which in turn will manufacture immune globulins. Proliferating plasma cells in association with malignancy of the plasmocytic system are not grouped around large mesenchymal cells.

The immunoglobulins manufactured by plasma cells produce many striking morphologic variants. The proteinaceous material is usually in the form of round, red globules called "Russell bodies" or "eosinophilic globules" (Plate 46). The globules do not always take the red stain but may be colorless or reveal pastel colors of pink, blue, or green. The globules may fill the cytoplasm, giving the appearance of a bunch of grapes (grape, berry, or morula cells). The secretory bodies are usually perfectly round (Plate 47).

In some cells, the spherules are so numerous and so tightly packed that they assume hexagonal or honey-comb shapes. In other cells, the fiery red color has a diffuse distribution, producing cells called "flame cells" or "flaming plasmocytes" (Plate 46). The red-staining material may appear as granules, as pools at the margins, or as extrusions through the cell membrane (Plate 46, Plate 47). After the escape of secretory products, the residual cytoplasmic stroma appears tattered and torn. The proteinaceous material within the cytoplasm may crystallize and produce elongated and pointed structures which may be colorless or stain various shades of red to purple (Plate 46). Rarely, there may be secretory globules of varying size and number in the nuclei (Plate 47).

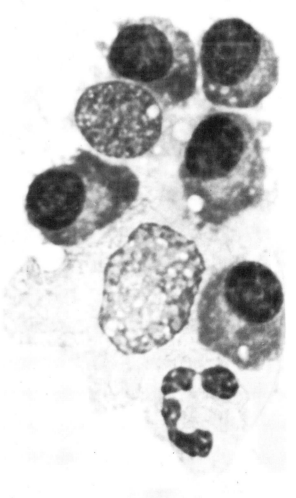

Fig 11—Plasmocytes clustered around finely granular tissue cells.

Plasmoblasts and Proplasmocytes. Blood cells designated as "plasmoblasts" are morphologically similar to the blastoid cells of other families of cells in that they are larger than the cells they are destined to produce. The nuclei are relatively large in relation to the cytoplasm. The cytoplasm is blue and nongranular. The nucleus is round and stains purplish-red. The chromatin strands are fine and linear. Nucleoli are clearly visible (Plate 7). The least-mature plasmoblast variants are differentiated from stem cells by association with other cells but cannot be differentiated from stem cells on the basis of size, shape, color, and structure. The more-mature plasmoblasts are more basophilic than the earlier forms due to the development of RNA particles which have an affinity for methylene blue.

Proplasmocytes and the most-mature plasma cells differ from plasmoblasts in that the color of the cytoplasm is dark blue, the juxtanuclear light areas are prominent, and the nuclei are eccentric. The nuclei of mature plasmocytes are pachychromatic, and the nucleoli are absent. The structure of the nuclei in proplasmocytes is intermediate between that of plasmoblasts and plasmocytes.

Malignancies involving Plasmocytes. Malignancies involving the cells of B cell lineage that are characterized by the proliferation of plasmocytes include Waldenstrom's disease, plasmocytoma, multiple myeloma, and plasma-cell leukemia.

Waldenstrom's disease (malignant macroglobulinemia) is a type of malignancy in which there is a mixture of B lymphocytes, plasmalike lymphocytes, and well-differentiated plasmocytes. These cells grow and multiply in multiple hematopoietic organs. The ratio of cells with morphologic characteristics of small lymphocytes and plasmocytes varies in different patients. Macroglobulin and blood viscosity increase. Rouleaux formation is marked.

Plasmocytomas are plasma-cell malignancies which, during their initial stages, are limited to focal areas in the bone marrow or in extramedullary areas.

Plasma-cell myelomas in their early stages are characterized by focal areas of proliferation in the bone marrow, followed by a progressive extension of growth in marrow spaces. Plasmocytes in small numbers are liberated into the blood. The plasmocytes vary in their morphologic characteristics (Fig 12). Mitotic figures and cells with multiple nuclei are demonstrable. There is asynchronism between nuclei and cytoplasm. Strands of precipitated globulin may be demonstrable in extracellular spaces. Rouleaux formation is a prominent feature.

Plasma-cell leukemia is a variant form of multiple myeloma characterized by the presence in the blood of large numbers of plasmocytic cells. Malignant plasmocytes are derived from stem cells and not from cells that morphologically resemble small lymphocytes (Fig 9, Fig 10, Fig 12).

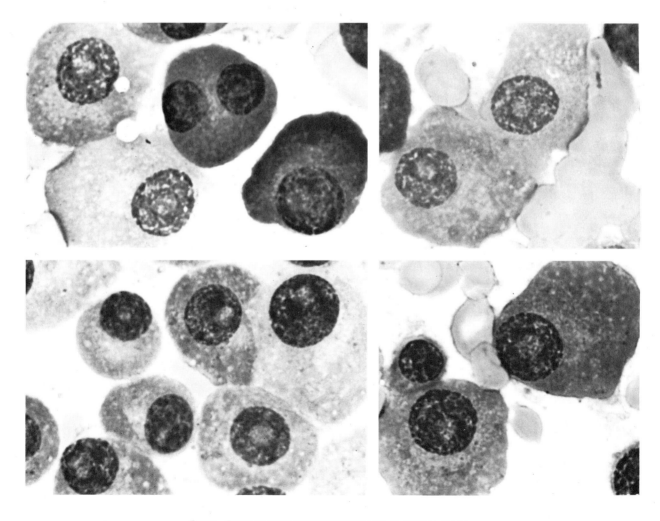

Fig 12—Plasmocytes in bone marrow smears, multiple myeloma.

Erythrocytes

ERYTHROPOIESIS. Mature erythrocytes are derived from committed erythroid progenitor cells through a series of mitotic divisions and maturation phases. Erythropoietin, a hormonal agent produced largely by the kidney, acts at the stem-cell level to induce proliferation and differentiation of erythrocytes. When anemia occurs and there is a change in the concentration of hemoglobin in the blood, there is a decrease in tissue oxygen within the kidney. Responding to this, the kidney produces erythropoietin which stimulates erythropoiesis and induces the erythroid stem cell to increase red-cell production, followed by increased blood oxygen-carrying capacity and increased tissue oxygen.

Erythropoiesis occurs in the marrow over a period of about five days through successive morphologic alterations from the rubriblast to a metarubricyte followed by a nonnucleated diffusely basophilic erythrocyte and later by a mature erythrocyte. During the early maturation period, mitochondria, Golgi apparatus, and polyribosomes are developed. Genes related to hemoglobin synthesis are activated, and in the cytoplasm of the later developmental stages, there is increasing hemoglobin synthesis. Three or four mitotic divisions occur in the early phases, but in the late phase, the cells are not able to divide.

The main functions of erythrocytes are to transport oxygen to the tissues and to return carbon dioxide to the lungs from the tissues. This gaseous exchange within the erythrocyte is facilitated by the oxygen-carrying protein, hemoglobin. The presence of hemoglobin usually is not visible as a reddish color in normal nucleated red cells until the rubricyte stage. In addition to hemoglobin, mature erythrocytes also contain enzymes for the production of energy and for maintenance of hemoglobin in the reduced state. Another function of erythrocytes is to maintain acid-base equilibrium.

Different terms are employed for red cells; synonyms in common use are given in Table 5.

Rubriblast. The earliest cells of the erythrocytic sequence are similar to other undifferentiated cells or "blasts." Nucleoli are usually visible. The chromatin strands are linear and distinct. In the very earliest forms, the cytoplasm stains a light blue, but in later and more frequently occurring forms, there is a superimposed reddish tint, due to the presence of hemoglobin, which imparts to the cytoplasm a peculiar dark and royal-blue color which is quite similar to that seen in certain plasmocytes (Plate 1D).

Prorubricyte. This cell is differentiated from the rubriblast by the coarsening of the chromatin pattern and ill-defined or absent nucleoli. The cytoplasm contains varying amounts of hemoglobin which has a reddish tinge, but the predominant color is blue (Plate 1D, Plate 8). Prorubricytes are normally smaller than rubriblasts.

Rubricyte. Rubricytes are smaller than prorubricytes, have relatively more cytoplasm, and take varying mixtures of red and blue stains. The nuclear chromatin is thickened and irregularly condensed, and nucleoli are no longer visible (Plate 1D, Plate 8).

Metarubricyte. The metarubricyte has a predominantly red cytoplasm and minimal amounts of residual blue. The nucleus is relatively small and has a nonlinear clumped chromatin structure or a solid blue-black degenerated nucleus (Plate 1D, Plate 8). Nucleated red cells with fragmented or partially extruded nuclei (Plate 18G) are classified as metarubricytes. The nucleus is extruded from the metarubricyte in the marrow, leaving a diffusely basophilic cell.

Diffusely Basophilic Erythrocyte. These cells have lost their nuclei but still maintain some of their bluish color (Plate 1, Plate 8) due to the presence of ribosomes (Plate 1D, Plate 8). They are larger than mature red cells. Diffusely basophilic cells, when stained with new methylene blue or other supravital dyes before they are fixed, reveal granulofilamentous structures and are identified as "reticulocytes." The diffusely basophilic cell is released in one to two days from the marrow and circulates in the peripheral blood and spleen for one to two days before maturing into an erythrocyte.

Erythrocyte. Normal erythrocytes are biconcave discs, 6 to 8 μm in diameter and 1.5 to 2.5 μm thick, which appear in stained smears as circular objects with distinct and smooth margins. The intensity of the stain in the central portion where the cell is thinnest is less than at the thicker marginal area (Plate 1D, Plate 8). In very thin coverslip preparations and

Table 5—Synonyms: Red Cells		
Rubriblast	Proerythroblast	Pronormoblast
Prorubricyte	Basophilic erythroblast Early erythroblast	Basophilic normoblast Early normoblast
Rubricyte	Polychromatophilic erythroblast Polychromatic erythroblast Intermediate erythroblast	Polychromatophilic normoblast Polychromatic normoblast Intermediate normoblast
Metarubricyte	Orthochromatic erythroblast Acidophilic erythroblast Normochromic erythroblast Late erythroblast	Orthochromatic normoblast Acidophilic normoblast Late normoblast
Diffusely basophilic erythrocyte	Polychromatophilic erythrocyte Polychromatic erythrocyte Proerythrocyte Reticulocyte	Reticulocyte
Erythrocyte	Erythrocyte	Erythrocyte

Left column: Macrocytic erythrocytes (megalocytic, megaloblastic) of the type seen in pernicious anemia and related B$_{12}$-folic acid deficient states

Middle column: Normal erythrocytic sequence

Right column: Microcytic, hypochromic cells of type seen in iron deficient states

Rubriblasts

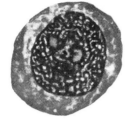 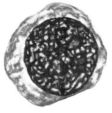 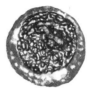

Prorubricytes

Rubricytes

Metarubricytes

Diffusely basophilic erythrocytes

Erythrocytes

PLATE 8—ERYTHROCYTIC SYSTEM

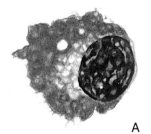 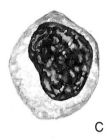 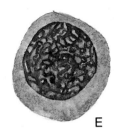

A   C   E

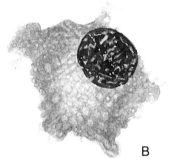 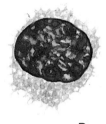 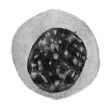

B   D   F

PLATE 9—COMPARATIVE MORPHOLOGY:
PLASMOCYTES, LYMPHOCYTES, AND IMMATURE NUCLEATED RED CELLS

A   Plasmocyte with intense-blue cytoplasm, eccentric nucleus, clear zone, vacuoles, and irregular shape

B   Plasmocyte with eccentric nucleus, foamy and fibrillar reddish-blue cytoplasm

C   Lymphocyte with slightly indented nucleus and unevenly stained bluish cytoplasm

D   Lymphocyte with foamy cytoplasm and frayed (hairlike) margins

E   Prorubricyte with reddish-blue cytoplasm

F   Rubricyte with polychromatophilia

at the extreme ends of smears, the red cells are flattened out like pancakes and do not reveal their true biconcave shapes. Very thin areas of smears where the erythrocytes are of uniform thickness are favorable for the visualization and identification of malarial parasites and other cytoplasmic objects but are unfavorable areas for the evaluation of hemoglobin concentration.

Nucleated Red Cells Clustered Around Phagocyte.
Tissue phagocytes that have acquired iron from ingested red blood cells and erythrocyte fragments serve as feeder or nursing cells to nucleated red cells that cluster around their margins (Fig 13). There is intimate intercellular contact between the satellite nucleated erythrocytes and the macrophage, with the phagocyte supplying nutrients, such as ferritin, to the surrounding nucleated cells, a process similar to nursing.

Prorubricytes vs. Plasmocytes vs. Lymphocytes.
Prorubricytes, plasmocytes and lymphocytes have in common a round nucleus without lobulations and a blue, nongranular cytoplasm (Plate 9). Plasmocytes and immature cells of the erythrocytic series may have mixtures of red and blue in their cytoplasm which gives them an intense royal-blue color. In iron-deficiency anemias, the rubricytes and metarubricytes are deficient in hemoglobin, and the blue color of the cytoplasm closely simulates that of lymphocytes. Lymphocytes as well as plasmocytes may have bubbly or foamy cytoplasm.

Prorubricytes do not have a bubbly cytoplasm or fibrillar structure, seldom contain vacuoles, and usually have smooth margins. They have less cytoplasm than plasmocytes, the perinuclear clear zone is less striking, and the nuclei are not eccentric (Plate 9).

Features which favor the diagnosis of the cell as a plasmocyte are the relatively large amount of cytoplasm, the oval shape, the eccentric nucleus, the relatively large light area next to the nucleus, the globules and vacuoles, the fibrillar structure, and the frayed edges (Plate 9).

Lymphocytes have a narrow rim of blue cytoplasm; the perinuclear clear zone is present, and the nucleus is not eccentric (Plate 9). Red color of the cytoplasm occasionally seen in plasma cells and in immature nucleated red cells is not present.

In many individual cells, the similarity between plasmocytes, prorubricytes, and lymphocytes is so close that differentiation cannot be made on morphologic grounds alone. Often it is necessary to classify the atypical cell by association with predominant cells or by arbitrarily placing it in the column statistically most likely. As in any other problem in differential morphology, a thin smear, a critical stain, a good microscope, a bright light, and experience are essential.

Pathological Erythrocytes.
The nucleated erythrocytes in marrow smears of patients with **pernicious anemia and related B$_{12}$-folic acid deficiency diseases** are larger than normal and demonstrate asynchronism between the nucleus and cytoplasm, with hemoglobin synthesized in advance of

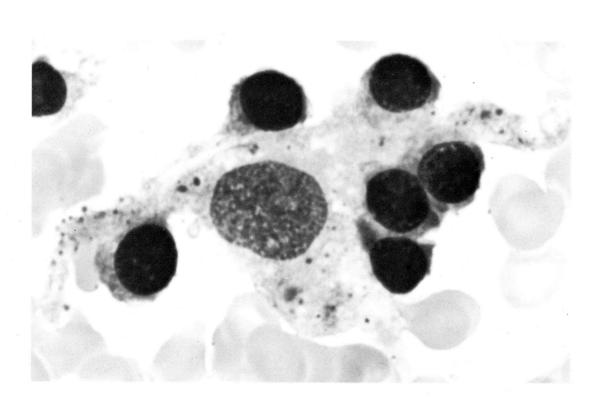

Fig 13—Nucleated red cells clustered around a tissue phagocyte.

the maturation of nuclear characteristics (Plate 18, Plate 27). The nuclei of the earliest cells reveal marked variation in chromatin structure. Some nuclei have delicate and uniformly distributed chromatin strands, while others may have lumpy as well as coarse linear chromatin patterns with wide separation between chromatin and parachromatin. Occasionally, there are slightly stained areas in the nucleus which are relatively devoid of chromatin. Nucleoli are usually demonstrable in the first and second stages of maturation.

The amount of cytoplasm in relation to the nucleus is increased. The color of the cytoplasm of the immature cells is intensely purplish-blue (Plate 18, Plate 27), making it difficult to differentiate the earliest stages. In some cells, small areas of reddish-staining hemoglobin shining through the basophilia are visible in the cytoplasm.

Increased numbers of mitotic figures in the immature erythroid cells are observed (Plate 27). Aberrant chromosomal fragments also may be present in the cytoplasm of cells in mitosis. Howell-Jolly bodies may be seen in the erythroid precursors.

Peripheral blood smears reveal variation in the size and shape of erythrocytes, with oval macrocytes and teardrop erythrocytes predominating (Plate 20). The mean corpuscular volume is increased (more than 100 fL or μm^3) due to the presence of numerous cells that are larger than normal. There are also microcytes and irregularly shaped cells that are smaller than normal. Diffusely basophilic cells are present. Other erythrocyte variants include macrocytic nucleated red cells with full hemoglobin component (Plate 18, Plate 27), Howell-Jolly bodies (Plate 18, Plate 27), nucleated red cells demonstrating karyorrhexis (Plate 18, Plate 27), and Cabot rings (Plate 18, Plate 27, Fig 16).

Immature nucleated erythrocytes observed in **anemias due to chronic blood loss** or to **nutritional deficiencies**, such as **iron deficiency** or in various types of **thalassemia** are smaller than normal, have a decreased amount of hemoglobin in their cytoplasm, and tend to have a relative increase in cytoplasmic basophilia in contrast to normal nucleated red cells. In severe iron deficiency, the small nucleated red cells have scanty blue-staining cytoplasm which has ragged edges. These small nucleated red cells observed in hemoglobin-deficient diseases may be confused with small lymphocytes. In addition to the morphologic changes, there is an erythroid hyperplasia in the marrow which varies depending on the degree of anemia.

The nucleated red cells in the smears of peripheral blood and bone marrow of patients with malignancies involving the erythrocytic cells, ie, **erythroleukemia**, reveal marked variation in size, shape, color, and structure and show asynchronism in nuclear and cytoplasmic development. There is variability in nuclear chromatin, with delicate chromatin strands in some cells and a clumped pattern in other cells. There may be aberrant nuclear masses. Vacuoles of varying size and shape appear often in the cytoplasm. There is intense erythroid hyperplasia of the marrow. The erythroblasts are distinctly abnormal, with giant cells, multinucleated forms, nuclear budding, and nuclear fragmentation (Plate 44, Plate 45). Mitotic figures are numerous and often bizarre. Periodic acid Schiff stain gives a coarse red granular positivity in the abnormal nucleated red cells, whereas normal nucleated erythrocytes are negative or show a faint diffuse reddish color.

The various maturation stages of dysplastic nucleated red cells from patients with abnormalities involving erythrocytes—such as pernicious anemia, microcytic hypochromic anemia, or erythroleukemia—should be categorized and reported by the standard nomenclature recommended by the College of American Pathologists. The classification should be "rubriblasts," "prorubricytes," "rubricytes," and "metarubricytes," followed by a description of the morphologic abnormalities that are revealed. The identification should be based mainly on the structure of the nucleus and not on the size or color of the cytoplasm.

Anisocytosis, Poikilocytosis, Anisochromia. Marked anisocytosis, poikilocytosis, and hypochromia are characteristic features of **thalassemia major** (Plate 20).

Spherocytes are densely stained red cells lacking in central pallor and with diameters less than normal-sized red cells (Plate 19, Plate 20). Spherocytes are the characteristic erythrocyte abnormality of hereditary spherocytosis. Similar cells may be seen in acquired immune hemolytic anemias, in patients who have been transfused, in hemolytic anemia due to oxidant drugs, and in patients with increased hemolysis secondary to a large spleen.

An **ovalocyte** or **elliptocyte** is an elongated cell with blunt ends (Plate 19, Plate 20). A few oval red cells may be observed in normal individuals. Small numbers of ovalocytes are observed in iron deficiency, thalassemia, sickled hemoglobinopathies, and other anemias. Ovalocytes occur in increased numbers in hereditary ovalocytosis. Oval cells vary from slightly oval or egg-shaped to long pencillike forms. Macrocytic ovalocytes are typical of megaloblastic anemia.

Erythrocytes containing sickle-cell hemoglobin (Hb S) undergo shape alterations when deoxygenated in sealed moist preparations and in moist preparations of blood mixed with reducing agents such as sodium metabisulfite. The soluble sickle-cell hemoglobin when deoxygenated becomes insoluble and polymerizes in the form of elongated and pointed crystal-like structures. These linear polymers distort the elastic membrane, producing multipointed, fanlike shapes (Plate 23). Cells assuming this shape are capable of immediately reverting to the disc shape when reoxygenated. Such cells are known as reversible sickle cells.

Erythrocytes that are identified as **sickle cells** in air-exposed blood smears have undergone transformation over an extended portion of time, causing their membranes to lose their elasticity and become permanently sickled. These cells are called irreversible sickle cells. Sickled red cells (drepanocytes, meniscocytes) are thin, elongated erythrocytes with a point at each end; have no central pallor; and may have oat, crescent, "L," "V," or "S" shapes (Plate 19, Plate 21). Sickle cells as a class are darker-than-normal red cells and may have corrugated surfaces. In rare instances, there are rectangular cells. Schizocytes of all types may be found. Sickled erythrocytes are observed in the blood smears in sickle-cell anemia and Hb S-thalassemia and in small numbers in Hb SC disease. Irreversible sickled cells are not observed in air-exposed smears of the sickle-cell trait under normal conditions.

A **target cell** (codocyte) has a central area of hemoglobin pigment surrounded by a relatively clear area and a peripheral rim of hemoglobin (Plate 19). There may be an extension of the peripheral rim of hemoglobin to the center of the cell. Target cells are common in thalassemia, sickle-cell anemia, Hb S-thalassemia, and other types of hemoglobinopathies.

Microangiopathic hemolytic anemias (thrombotic thrombocytopenic purpura, uremia with hypertension, sickle-cell anemia with pulmonary emboli, diffuse intravascular coagulation, heart-valve prosthesis, disseminated carcinoma, and hemolytic uremic syndrome) are characterized by a variety of membrane-injured red cells including helmet, burr, acanthocyte, spur, spiculated, fragmented, pinched, and triangular and cells with marginal achromia (Plate 19, Plate 21, Fig 14).

There are marked changes in size, shape, and color in the erythrocytes in patients with extensive **burns** and with **hereditary pyropoikilocytosis** (Plate 22). The red cells in hereditary pyropoikilocytosis show striking fragmentation when heated to 45 °C in contrast to normal red cells which fragment at a higher temperature (49 °C).

The size and shape changes observed in **myelofibrosis** are shown in Plate 22.

Erythrocyte Inclusions. **Granulofilamentous material** (Plate 24) is visible in erythrocytes in supravital stain without preliminary fixation. The reticulated material is thought to consist of aggregated masses of RNA and possible degenerated mitochondria. Red cells containing this granular and filamentous network are called **reticulocytes**. Most cells identified as reticulocytes have lost their nuclei, but a rare metarubricyte with granulofilamentous material may be observed.

Reticulocytes in a supravital stain, such as new methylene blue, correspond to the diffusely basophilic cells appearing in Wright stain which contains methyl alcohol as a fixative (Fig 15). A count of reticulocytes indicates the physiologic activity of the marrow. Normal blood contains less than 2%. An increase in reticulocytes is observed in hemolytic anemia and after treatment for nutritional deficiencies. Decreased reticulocytes are seen in hypoplastic states.

Basophilic stippling in red cells represents aggregation of ribosomes which stain deep blue with Wright stain. This precipitated RNA appears as granules of varying sizes which are distributed throughout the cell (Plate 24, Fig 15). Stippling as revealed in Wright stain and the granulofilamentous network in supravital stain are related phenomena. Coarse basophilic stippling and increased reticulocytes are noted in lead or other heavy-metal intoxication and thalassemia. Stippled cells and increased reticulocytes also may be seen after treatment for nutritional deficiencies and after the use of cytotoxic drugs.

Howell-Jolly bodies are spherical nuclear fragments composed of DNA (Plate 18, Plate 27, Fig 15) which may be observed in erythrocytes on a blood film stained with Wright stain or with a supravital stain. Usually only one Howell-Jolly body is seen in a red cell. Normally, these nuclear remnants are pitted from erythrocytes during passage through the spleen. Howell-Jolly bodies are found in megaloblastic anemia, sickle-cell anemia, other hemolytic anemias, and hyposplenism and after splenectomy.

Cabot rings (Plate 18, Plate 27, Fig 16) are usually seen in the form of rings, but they also may appear as granules in a linear array rather than as complete rings. A ring may occur near the membrane, appearing to outline the cell, or make a figure-eight form. Rarely there may be more than one ring per red cell. These structures are frequently observed in stippled red cells, and they may also reside in the cytoplasm of nucleated red cells.

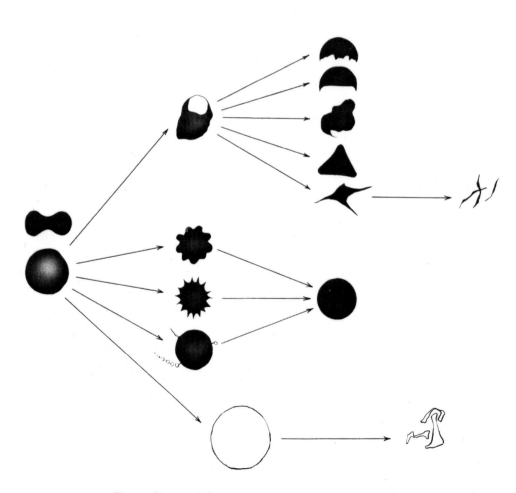

Fig 14—Shape variations in erythrocytes due to membrane alterations.

Megakaryocytes and Thrombocytes

CELLS OF THE MEGAKARYOCYTIC SYSTEM are peculiar in that the nucleus undergoes multiple mitotic divisions without cytoplasmic separation, thus producing giant polyploid cells (Plate 10, Plate 11). All the nuclei in a given cell undergo mitosis at the same time (Plate 11) producing two, four, eight, or—in rare instances—16 or 32 nuclei. The multiple nuclei usually remain attached to each other and are often superimposed, giving a lobular appearance. The dividing nuclei maintain the distinct linear chromatin pattern of young cells while the cytoplasm undergoes maturation changes characterized by the development of granules and membranes, culminating in platelet differentiation and liberation.

Well-defined platelet masses usually appear at the margins of megakaryocytes in the four to eight nucleate stages of development, but in some cells, platelets form in cells with single or double nuclei. When the nuclei and the cytoplasm are out of step with each other, it is recommended that the identity of the individual cell be established by the characteristics of the cytoplasm rather than by the chromatin structure or the number of nuclei. This is a departure from the rule that the structure of the nucleus is the most reliable criterion for identification.

Intact megakaryocytes, fragments of megakaryocytes, and naked nuclei are occasionally demonstrable in smears of peripheral blood from patients with myeloproliferative diseases such as chronic myelocytic and megakaryocytic leukemia and in leukemic myelofibrosis. They are seldom observed in peripheral blood smears of normal individuals. In bone marrow smears and in sections of marrow tissue from normal individuals, the megakaryocytes constitute one to four per 1,000 nucleated cells. Most of the megakaryocytic cells are in the third and fourth stages of maturation.

Megakaryoblast. The megakaryoblast is a large, irregularly shaped cell with a single nucleus or with several round or oval nuclei and with a blue, nongranular cytoplasm. There may be blunt pseudopods which stain various shades of blue and which may contain multiple chromophobic globules (Plate 10, Plate 11). Spongy ectoplasm of this type is often demonstrable in sarcoma and in other malignant cells but is not present or is inconspicuous in primitive cells of the erythrocytic or leukocytic series of blood cells. The nuclear chromatin strands in megakaryoblasts are distinct. Nucleoli usually are demonstrable (Plate 10).

Promegakaryocyte. The promegakaryocyte differs from the megakaryoblast in that there are bluish granules in the cytoplasm adjacent to the nucleus. The nucleus in this second stage of maturation has usually divided one or more times, and the cell has increased in size. Often there are bluish cytoplasmic extensions with rounded contours which may have a homogeneous or a bubbly appearance (Plate 10, Plate 11).

One of the variants of the promegakaryocyte is a cell with one or more nuclei with granular cytoplasm adjacent to the nucleus encircled by a collar of vacuolated cytoplasm and by a third and distinct marginal zone characterized by dark-blue and rounded cytoplasmic protrusions which stain unevenly and often contain small colorless globules (Plate 11).

Megakaryocyte (Megakaryocyte without thrombocytes). Megakaryocytic cells in the third stage of maturation are large cells with relatively large amounts of cytoplasm, round shapes, even margins, and multiple nuclei. The chromatin pattern of the nucleus is linear and coarse with distinct spaces between the chromatin strands. The cytoplasm contains numerous small, rather uniformly distributed granules which have a reddish-blue hue (Plate 10). Light-staining areas may be demonstrable.

Metamegakaryocyte (Megakaryocyte with thrombocytes). Megakaryocytic cells in the fourth stage of maturation are characterized by the aggregation of granular cytoplasmic material into masses which are separated from each other by relatively clear spaces (demarcation membranes or vesicles). These units of granular cytoplasm tend to aggregate near the periphery of the cell (Plate 10).

Megakaryocytes in the more-advanced stages of maturation are slowly ameboid. They extend portions of their cytoplasm through the basement membranes and between the endothelial cells of the sinusoids of the bone marrow. From these cytoplasmic protrusions, the differentiated and membrane-bound platelets separate and are swept into the flowing blood stream. Other megakaryocytes escape into the vascular channels of the marrow and are transported by veins to the lungs where they lodge in the terminal pulmonary arterioles and alveolar capillaries. From these sites, they continue to differentiate and to liberate portions of their cytoplasm in the form of platelets (Plate 10). The naked nuclei disintegrate or are phagocytized.

Thrombocyte (Platelet). Thrombocytes are fragments of cytoplasm of megakaryocytes. In spreads of blood from normal individuals, the diameters of individual platelets vary from 1 to 4 μm, but in various diseases, the size may range from barely visible structures to masses larger than red cells or leukocytes (Plate 36, Plate 50). As a rule, thrombocytes have

Table 6 — Morphological Features of Cells of the Megakaryocytic Series				
STATE OF MATURATION	CYTOPLASMIC GRANULES	THROMBOCYTES	CYTOPLASMIC TAGS	NUCLEAR CHARACTERISTICS
Megakaryoblast	Absent	Absent	Present	Single Fine chromatin structure Nucleoli
Promegakaryocyte	Few	Absent	Present	Double
Megakaryocyte	Numerous	Absent	Usually absent	Two or more nuclei
Metamegakaryocyte	Aggregated	Present	Absent	Four or more nuclei

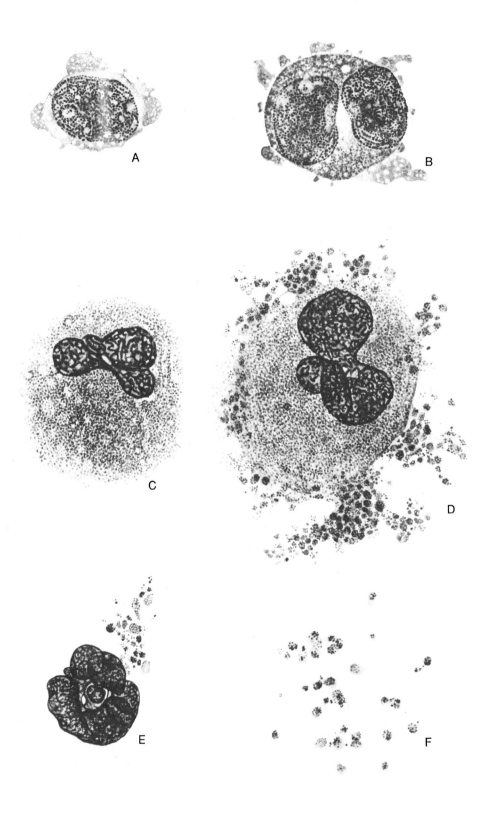

PLATE 10—MEGAKARYOCYTIC SYSTEM

A Megakaryoblast with single oval nucleus,
   nucleoli, and bluish foamy marginal
   cytoplasmic structures
B Promegakaryocyte with two nuclei, granular
   blue cytoplasm, and marginal bubbly
   cytoplasmic structures
C Megakaryocyte with granular cytoplasm and
   without discrete thrombocytes (platelets)

D Metamegakaryocyte with multiple nuclei and
   with thrombocytes (platelets)
E Metamegakaryocyte nucleus with attached
   thrombocytes
F Thrombocytes (platelets)

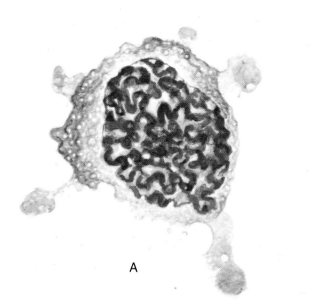

A

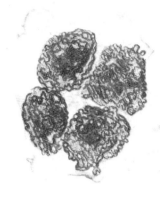

B

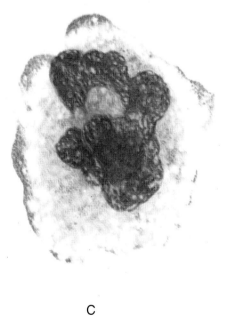

C

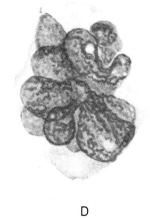

D

PLATE 11—MEGAKARYOCYTIC VARIANTS

A Megakaryoblast, in prophase
B Promegakaryocyte with four nuclei,
   beginning granule formation adjacent to nucleus,
   and blunt nongranular pseudopods

C Promegakaryocyte or intermediate
   megakaryocyte with multiple attached nuclei,
   granular cytoplasm surrounded by a ring of coarsely
   vacuolated cytoplasm and outer marginal darker
   blue zone, and no well-delineated thrombocytes
D Atypical promegakaryocyte with
   asynchronism between cytoplasm and nuclei,
   multiple attached superimposed nuclei, fine
   granules adjacent to nucleus, and nongranular
   ectoplasm.

multiple pointed filaments or tentaclelike protrusions (Plate 10). Round, oval, spindle, and discoid shapes with smooth margins are also observed. The cytoplasm stains a light blue and contains variable numbers of small, blue granules which tend to aggregate in the center (granulomere, chromomere) as contrasted with the marginal zone which is nongranular (hyalomere).

Platelets tend to adhere to each other (Plate 2). Individual platelets and clumps of platelets are most numerous at the distal (feather) ends of blood smears. In thin portions where the erythrocytes and leukocytes are well separated, the number per oil-immersion field varies from seven to 25. The number of platelets in the average oil-immersion field multiplied by 20,000 gives the approximate number per cubic millimeter. No report of a blood smear is complete unless the platelet number is stated and morphological abnormalities are described.

Platelets may appear as satellites around the cytoplasm of neutrophils when the blood smear is made with an anticoagulant, particularly ethylenediaminetetraacetic acid (EDTA) (Fig 18).

Morphological Abnormalities. The size of megakaryocytes is increased in association with a deficiency of B_{12} and/or folic acid. Large megakaryocytes usually have an increased number of nuclei (hyperlobulation). Small megakaryocytes (micromegakaryocytes) may be demonstrable in smears of bone marrow of patients with myelocytic and myelocytic-monocytic leukemia and in blast crisis of chronic granulocytic leukemia. These cells usually have a single round nucleus. The cytoplasm may contain fine bluish granules. As a rule, there are blunt marginal nongranular protrusions which vary in the intensity of their staining qualities (Plate 51). Platelet differentiation may be seen in these cells.

In idiopathic thrombocytopenic purpura, there is a relative and absolute increase in naked nuclei and in the number of megakaryocytes with granular cytoplasm and smooth margins.

The size and shape of platelets in thrombocytopenic states is variable (Plate 50). Giant platelets are demonstrable in the blood of patients with the May-Hegglin syndrome (Plate 36), leukemic myelofibrosis (Plate 50), thrombasthenia (Plate 50), and myeloproliferative diseases (Fig 19). Giant platelets also are increased after splenectomy.

Some of the large platelets contain aggregates of granular and linear material (granulomere) which sharply contrast with the nongranular peripheral areas (hyalomere) (Plate 50). Round or oval granular areas which stain more darkly than the other portions superficially resemble nuclei (Plate 50, Fig 19). These aggregates differ from nuclei in that their margins are irregular and there is an absence of nuclear membrane.

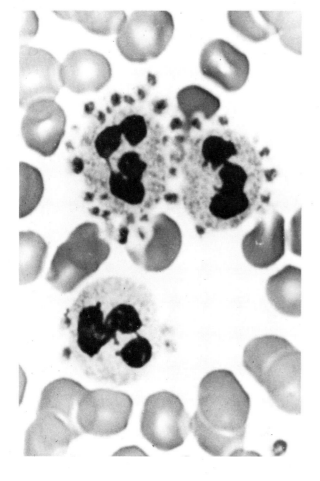

Fig 18—Photomicrograph of platelet satellitosis.

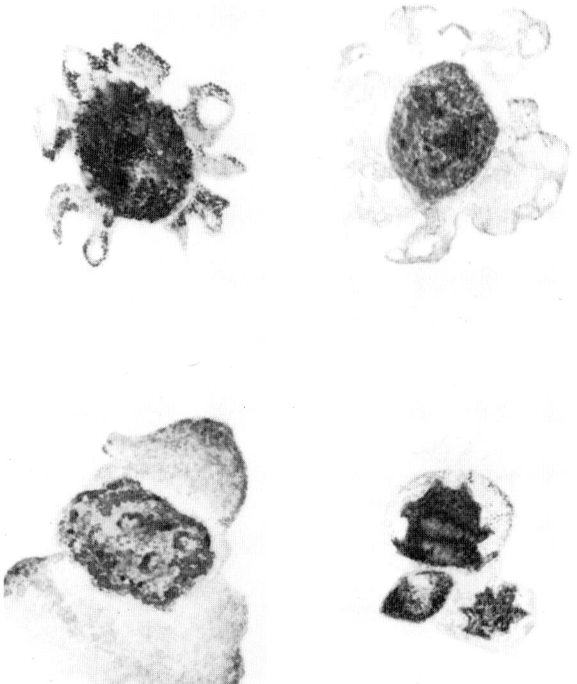

Fig 19—Drawing of platelets; myelofibrosis.

FIXED
TISSUE
CELLS

FREE
BLOOD
CELLS

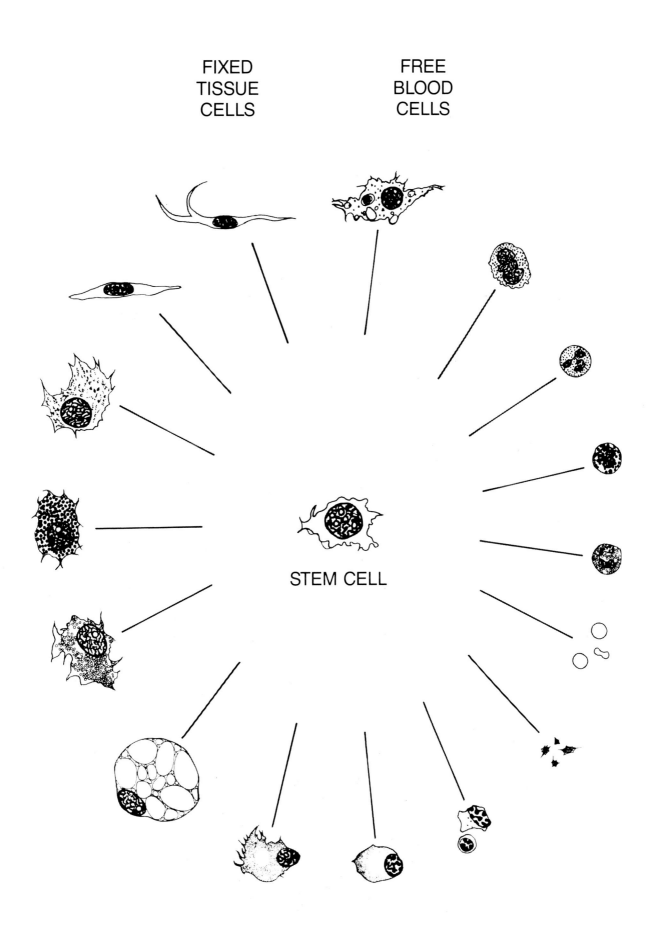

STEM CELL

Fig 20—Fixed tissue cells and free blood cells originating
from totipotent stem cell.

III TISSUE CELLS

IN ADDITION to the free blood cells of the peripheral blood and their precursors in the bone marrow, there are various types of fixed tissue cells. These cells are relatively immobile and are attached to other cells or imbedded by their cytoplasmic extensions in the ground substance of the marrow and entrapped within the network of reticular and collagen fibers. They are aspirated with difficulty and are best seen in tissue sections.

Stained tissue sections of bone marrow supplement the examination of marrow smears by revealing the degree of cellularity and fibrosis and the relationship of marrow cells to fat, trabecular bone, and blood vessels. Tissue sections also provide information about the number of megakaryocytes, tissue basophils, and giant cells, as well as the presence or absence of hemorrhage, degenerative and necrotic lesions, granulomas, and amyloid and malignant cells.

Stem Cells

STEM CELLS are morphologically undifferentiated cells that are progenitors of blood and tissue cells of various types (Plate 13, Plate 14, Plate 54, Fig 20). Stem cells are capable of self-replication, thus making it possible to maintain ancestral cells that are readily available to replace cells that are lost from, or destroyed in, the body. Some of the cells of the stem-cell pool, after appropriate stimulation, produce cells with distinctive functional and anatomical characteristics.

Stem cells are not demonstrable in the peripheral blood of normal individuals. Stem cells are identified in blood smears only in association with malignancies involving the blood-forming organs. The number of stem cells in bone marrow in the absence of myeloproliferative diseases is less than one per 1,000 nucleated cells.

The size of stem cells is variable, depending on their nutrition and their growth between mitotic divisions. The cells that are identified and reported as stem cells are the larger forms (Plate 14). Small stem cells are likely to be mistakenly identified as lymphocytes.

Since stem cells in the bone marrow are fixed tissue cells that are mechanically traumatized in the process of aspiration, these cells usually have irregular shapes, frayed margins, and blunt cytoplasmic projections (Plate 14).

The nuclei of stem cells are round or oval. The chromatin strands are fine and linear. The nuclear substance between the chromatin threads (parachromatin) is well defined. There is no evidence of chromatin clumping. Several nucleoli which stain light blue usually are demonstrable.

The cytoplasm of stem cells may contain a few indistinct purplish granules. There are no large and well-defined granules. There is no evidence of phagocytic particles or digestive vacuoles. The color of the cytoplasm is light blue.

Stem cells as a class contain in their cytoplasm fewer RNA bodies than cells designated as "blasts." Cells that are precursors of "blasts" therefore stain less-intensely blue than typical blasts. Fine differences in shades of blue, however, are difficult to discern, are impossible to define, and vary depending on the stain and the staining technique employed.

In the process of counting and reporting the percentage of nucleated cells of various types, it is recommended that morphologically undifferentiated cells with round nuclei, delicate nuclear chromatin strands, nucleoli, and nongranular blue cytoplasm be reported as "stem cells" if they are present in small numbers. On the other hand, if the anaplastic cells are associated with large numbers of definitive cells and if transitional forms are readily demonstrable, the cells that are difficult to identify are categorized as blast cells of the clone that is predominent. For example, in smears of blood or bone marrow of patients with myelocytic leukemia, the undifferentiated cells are identified as "myeloblasts." Undifferentiated cells demonstrable in a patient with lymphocytic leukemia are called "lymphoblasts," etc. In marrow smears from normal individuals or from patients with diseases in which the diagnosis is not possible, cells with nonspecific anatomical features are reported as "stem cells" rather than "blasts." In leukemic states in which all of the blood cells are morphologically and functionally immature, the diagnosis of "stem cell leukemia" is justified.

Nucleated cells that are identified in hematopoietic organs as stem cells may be progenitors of fixed tissue cells as well as of free blood cells (Fig 20). Totipotent cells that have the capability of developing into hemic, as well as tissue, cells have been designated as "hemohistioblasts." Stem cells that are presumed to be precursors of blood cells *only* have been called "hemocytoblasts." The term "immunoblast" has been employed by some to designate cells that are thought to be destined to produce progeny that are immunologically competent. These terms relate to concepts and theories rather than to morphologic entities. It is not possible by looking at a given anaplastic cell to predict the appearance or the function of the daughter cells that will be produced by that cell. Tissue cells with nonspecific structural characteristics should be reported as "unclassified" and should not be identified as "reticuloendothelial cells" or as "reticulum cells."

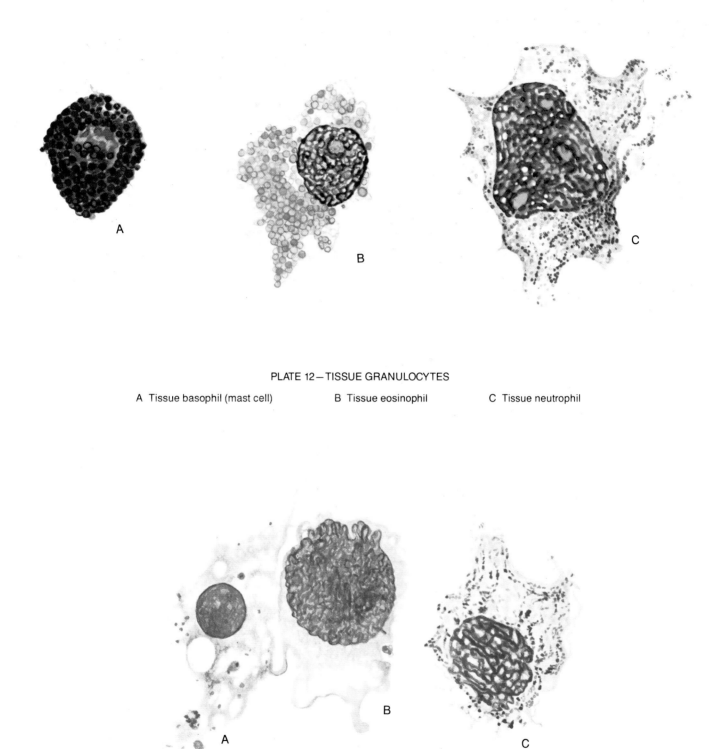

PLATE 12—TISSUE GRANULOCYTES

A Tissue basophil (mast cell)   B Tissue eosinophil   C Tissue neutrophil

PLATE 13—FIXED TISSUE CELLS

A Phagocytic histiocyte with vacuoles and
   phagocytized malarial pigment
B Stem cell with partial rupture of
   nuclear membrane and blue
   nongranular cytoplasm

C Tissue neutrophil with coarse nuclear chromatin
   structure, neutrophilic granules, and shaggy
   margins

Tissue Granulocytes

TISSUE GRANULOCYTES of the basophilic, eosinophilic, and neutrophilic types are derived from stem cells. Early tissue granulocytes lack distinctive characteristics. Tissue granulocytes are thought to be end-stage cells that do not differentiate into mature and motile granulocytes (Fig 20).

Tissue Basophils (Mast cells, heparinocytes). Tissue basophils are fixed tissue cells that are traumatized in the process of aspiration and therefore often have jagged margins. Many of the cells have spindle shapes and oval nuclei. The size varies. As a rule, the diameters of the more-round tissue basophils are from two to four times those of red cells in the same field. The nucleus is relatively small and is round or oval. The cytoplasm is filled with intensely stained violet-blue granules. The granules are uniformly round and are approximately the same size (0.1 to 0.3 μm). They frequently overlie the margins of the relatively pale nucleus or may partially or completely obscure the nucleus (Plate 12A, Fig 21).

Tissue basophils are widely scattered in various organs including the bone marrow. They usually are not encountered while performing a differential count of a few hundred cells but may be relatively increased and conspicuous in conditions associated with pancytopenia and myelosclerosis. Mast cells may proliferate as localized tumors (urticaria pigmentosa) or as a systemic disease (systemic mastocytosis).

Tissue basophils and blood basophils are closely related in their chemical characteristics and in their functions. Their difference is mainly one of motility.

Blood Basophils vs Tissue Basophils. Opinions differ about the relationship of actively motile blood basophils and basophils that reside as slowly ameboid or fixed cells in connective-tissue areas of various organs. The granules of blood and tissue basophils have similar morphologic characteristics. The granules in both types of basophils are water soluble and are metachromatic. The granules in both types of cells contain heparin and histamine.

The heparin secreted by perivascular tissue cells and by blood basophils aids in preventing intravascular coagulation and in maintaining the fluidity of the blood. There usually is an associated hemorrhagic tendency in diseases characterized by an increase in basophilic cells in the bone marrow.

Blood basophils as well as tissue basophils participate in a similar manner in acute and in delayed allergic reactions. After release of histamine, the manifestations include increased vascular permeability, perivascular edema, increased secretion of fluid from mucous membranes, and itching. A massive and systemic release of histamine from basophilic granules, as with the bites of wasps or the injection of serum or a drug to which the individual is highly sensitive, may lead to bronchospasm, edema of the respiratory tract, anaphylactic shock, and sudden death.

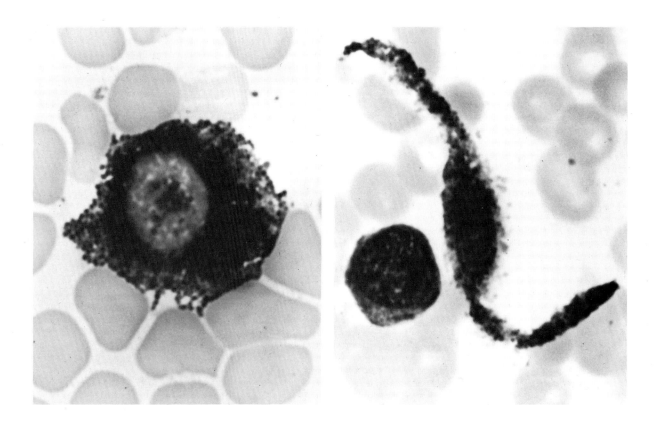

Fig 21—Tissue basophils.

Tissue Eosinophils. In smears of bone marrow, one occasionally sees large cells with elongate and tapering cytoplasmic extensions and containing typical red granules of the type seen in the eosinophils of the circulating blood. The nuclei of such cells, instead of being indented or lobulated, resemble those of the other fixed tissue cells, being round or oval and having well-defined reticular chromatin patterns and often nucleoli (Plate 12B, Fig 22).

It is thought that tissue eosinophils are fixed tissue variants of the more motile eosinophils of the circulating blood.

Tissue Neutrophils (Ferrata cells). One of the cell types, which is encountered in small numbers (less than 1%) in practically every smear of normal bone marrow, is a cell which resembles the undifferentiated mesenchymal cell except for the fact that it contains varying numbers of neutrophilic granules.

Tissue neutrophils are large with ample cytoplasm. In rare instances, one may find a round or oval variant with smooth contours, but as a rule, the shape is bizarre, with a combination of blunt pseudopods and multipointed and nebulous cytoplasmic streamers. These cells are readily indented by adjacent cells or are squeezed in between them (Fig 23, Fig 24). Often there are long and tenuous cytoplasmic extensions which seem to wrap around other cells. These cells are not phagocytic and seldom have vacuoles in the cytoplasm.

The cytoplasm stains light blue and has a fine latticelike structure (Plate 12C, Plate 13C, Plate 14D). Granules vary in number. The granules stain varying shades of red to blue, but the majority take a brilliant red or reddish-purple stain. Many of the granules tend to be arranged in chains. The beadlike aggregates extend into the cytoplasmic projections where they tend to be parallel to each other and to the cytoplasmic margins (Plate 12C).

The large round or oval nucleus has a coarse chromatin structure with a distinct linear pattern. Nucleoli are usually conspicuous (Plate 12C).

Tissue neutrophils (Ferrata cells) are increased in bone marrow smears in conditions in which there is proliferation of neutrophilic cells. These cells may be prominent in bone marrow smears in myelocytic and monomyelocytic leukemia (Naegeli type of monocytic leukemia), in leukemic myelosis, in pernicious anemia, and in conditions in which there is injury to cells associated with maturation arrest and a neutropenic state due to chemicals and cytotoxic agents. Tissue neutrophils may be demonstrable in the peripheral blood of patients with myelocytic or monomyelocytic leukemia.

Many hematologists have assumed, and hematology texts often have stated, that large neutrophilic granulocytes with irregular shapes that are demonstrable in bone marrow smears and that are designated as "Ferrata cells" are squashed promyelocytes and myelocytes. It is true that degenerated and mashed immature neutrophils superficially resemble tissue neutrophils, but this is not an indication that well-preserved tissue neutrophils are artifacts. The demonstration of mitotic figures in cells that have the cytoplasmic and nuclear characteristics of tissue neutrophils is proof that these cells are not senile and degenerative variants.

It is universally accepted that there are fixed tissue basophils and tissue eosinophils (Plate 12), as well as free basophils and eosinophils, tissue phagocytes, motile monocytes and macrophages, and tissue plasmocytes. There also are circulating plasmocytes. Thus it is reasonable to assume that tissue neutrophils are not artifacts.

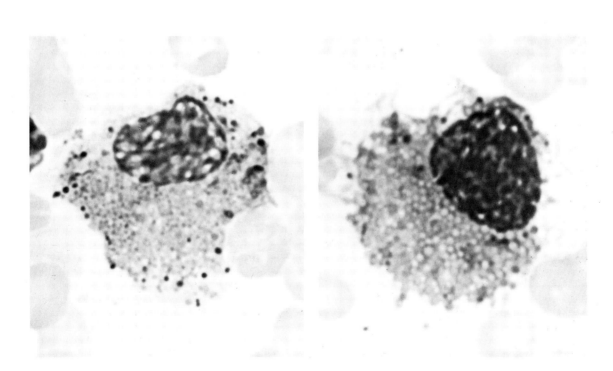

Fig 22—Tissue eosinophils.

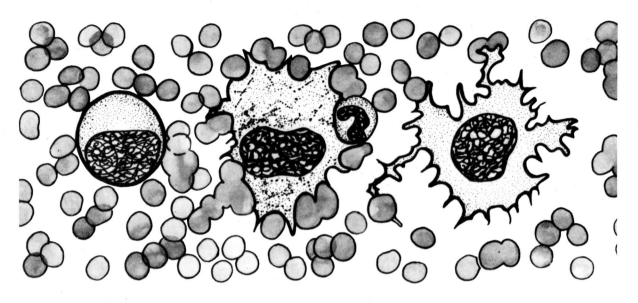

N. MYELOCYTE　　　TISSUE NEUTROPHIL　　　HAIRY CELL

Fig 23 — Relationship of myelocyte, tissue neutrophil, and
hairy cell to surrounding cells.

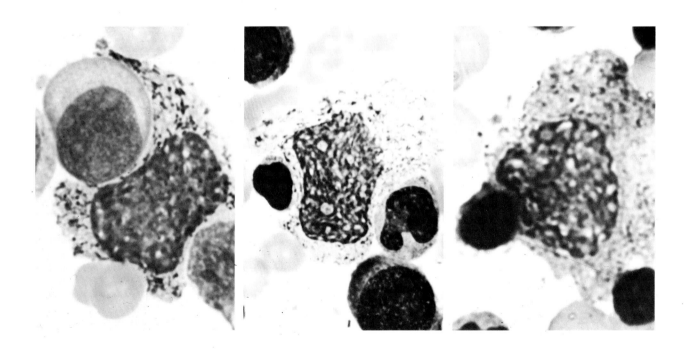

Fig 24 — Tissue neutrophils (Ferrata cells).

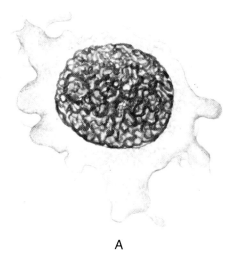

A

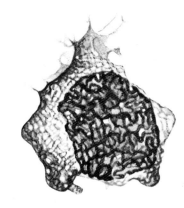

B

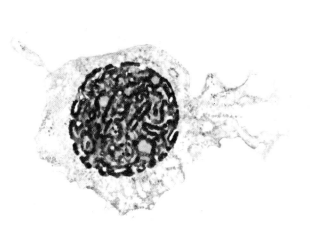

C

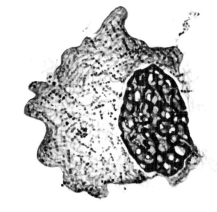

D

PLATE 14—FIXED TISSUE CELLS

A,B Undifferentiated mesenchymal cell
(hemohistioblast, stem cell) with irregular
shape, blue cytoplasm with no granules,
linear chromatin, and nucleoli

C Unclassified immature fixed tissue cell with
minimal granulation, fibrillar structure, and
cytoplasmic extensions

D Tissue neutrophil with few granules

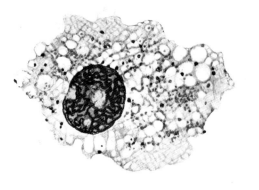

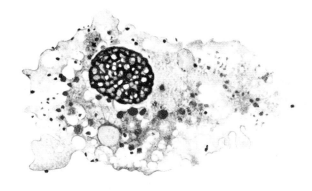

A B

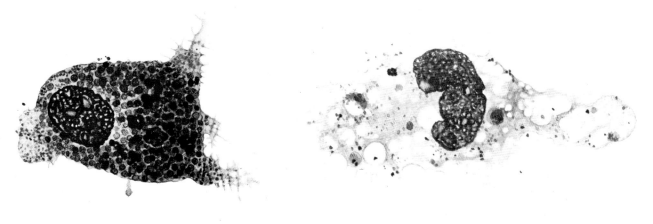

C D

PLATE 15—MACROPHAGES

A Phagocytic histiocyte with reticular cytoplasmic
structure, vacuoles, and phagocytized particles

B Phagocytic histiocyte (ameboid macrophage)
with phagocytized erythrocytes and dark-
staining particles

C Phagocytic histiocyte, fixed tissue type with
phagocytized hemosiderin in cytoplasm

D Ameboid phagocyte (wandering
tissue macrophage) with phagocytized particles
and vacuoles in cytoplasm

Macrophages (Tissue Phagocytes, Phagocytic Histiocytes)

BLOOD CELLS designated as "macrophages" are large mononuclear cells that are capable of phagocytizing particulate matter. These cells, during postnatal life, originate in the bone marrow from progenitor cells designated as "monoblasts." After maturation in marrow spaces, monocytes escape into the blood where they function as phagocytic cells. Some of these motile cells squirm between endothelial-lining cells of terminal blood vessels and through basement membranes of vascular channels into perivascular connective-tissue spaces where their growth continues. Some of these cells attach to connective-tissue fibers and become fixed. Other macrophages fulfill their function as wandering tissue cells.

Fixed tissue cells that have phagocytic properties and are known as "Kupffer cells" are interspersed with endothelial-lining cells in the sinusoids of the liver. Other tissue phagocytes are demonstrable in the spleen, lymph nodes, and bone marrow and in small numbers in the connective-tissue spaces of all other organs.

Macrophages, as the name implies, are large cells. The diameters of these cells are two to four times those of neutrophils in the same microscopic fields. The more-motile cells are usually elongated and reveal blunt pseudopods (Plate 15). The more-fixed tissue phagocytes that are torn away from their moorings at the time of aspiration have shaggy margins and multiple tapering cytoplasmic protrusions.

The nuclei are relatively small in relation to the cytoplasm. They are round, oval, or slightly indented. The chromatin pattern is linear. Nucleoli often are demonstrable.

The cytoplasm of macrophages stains light blue and has a fine reticular structure. There are numerous granules of varying sizes (Plate 15). Vacuoles are demonstrable in the cytoplasm of most of the cells. Phagocytized objects that may be revealed in digestive vacuoles include intact red cells (Plate 15) and leukocytes, cell fragments, platelets, hemosiderin (Plate 15), bacteria, fungi (Plate 53, left), protozoa (Plate 53, right), and crystals.

Mononuclear microphages (monocytes) as well as occasional mononuclear macrophages are demonstrable in all types of body fluids including urine, sputum, saliva, tears, cerebrospinal fluid, and mucous secretions from the nose and facial sinuses. Phagocytic monocytic cells also are demonstrable in the secretions of the gastrointestinal and genital tracts, in serous and synovial fluids, and in transudates and exudates. The sputum of patients with congestive heart failure and stasis of blood in pulmonary vessels contains macrophages laden with hemosiderin (heart-failure cells).

Mononuclear phagocytes of the tissue spaces acquire antigen from ingested microorganisms, from cells that are foreign to the body, and from chemicals bound to proteins that have antigenic properties. The acquired antigens are processed in the macrophages. Templates of these antigenic substances are transferred to lymphocytes and plasmocytes that cluster around the margins of the central phagocytes (Fig 11). After stimulation by antigenic material supplied by central feeder cells, the satellite cells transform into cells that become immunologically effective.

Lipid-Storage Diseases (Lipoidoses). Cells of the monocyte-macrophage system phagocytize and digest cell fragments and degenerated and dead cells of all types. When there are inherited deficiencies in the production of enzymes necessary for the catabolism of ingested cells, lipids of various types—depending on the type of enzyme that is lacking—accumulate in the cytoplasm of the phagocytic cells. Diseases associated with the storage of greasy and waxy structures (lipids) are designated as "lipid-storage diseases" or as "lipoidoses."

There are numerous types of storage diseases. From a hematological point of view, Gaucher's and Neimann-Pick's diseases are of particular interest because the fat-laden macrophages in these diseases are numerous and are readily demonstrable in bone marrow smears and tissue sections.

The cytoplasmic inclusions in the macrophages of patients with Gaucher's disease are glucocerebrosides. **Gaucher cells** (Plate 52, left) are large with irregular shapes. They usually occur as grouped fixed tissue cells. The nuclei are round and relatively small. The chromatin strands are distinct. Multiple nuclei may be demonstrable. The pale-blue cytoplasm is stuffed with doubly refractile and membrane-bound tubular structures of varying lengths. Cells that contain short tubules have a finely granular ground-glass appearance. The most characteristic cells have a linear or fibrillar appearance due to the presence of elongated and narrow lipid inclusions. Some of the rodlike structures are bent and have tapered ends (crescentric or sicklelike shapes). Chromophobic tubular structures that overlie or underlie the nucleus may be demonstrable. Apt descriptive terms that have been used include "wrinkled cellophane," "crumpled tissue paper," and "crinkled silk."

Lipid-laden macrophages with elongated chromophobic cytoplasmic inclusions may be demonstrable in small numbers in bone marrow of patients with diseases other than Gaucher's disease. These cells are designated as "**pseudo-Gaucher cells**." Gaucher-like cells may be demonstrable in the bone marrow of patients with chronic myeloid leukemia and in numerous other diseases. The inclusions that are present in non-Gaucher cells are explained by the fact that dead cells are phagocytized at a rate faster than the lipids in these cells can be digested.

Cytoplasmic lipid inclusions of the Neimann-Pick type are due to accumulations of sphingomyelin that cannot be degraded and disposed of because there is a deficiency in the enzyme necessary for the breakdown and disposal. **Neimann-Pick cells** are large with relatively small round nuclei. The cytoplasm is filled with small chromophobic and spherical inclusions enclosed by blue-staining fibrils (Plate 52, right). The fat globules in Neimann-Pick cells differ from the globules of fat in lipocytes in the bone marrow of normal individuals in that they are uniformly small and spherical. The globules of normal cells, in contrast, vary in size and shape (Plate 16).

Phagocytic cells that have a foamy or bubbly cytoplasm and reticular stromal pattern are demonstrable as isolated or as grouped cells in the bone marrow of patients with numerous diseases. The presence of tissue cells with multiple small digestive vacuoles is a nonspecific manifestation of cytoplasmic overloading. The presence of large numbers of cells with prominent chromophobic cytoplasmic inclusions should alert the examiner to the possibility of lipoidoses in which there is a gene-determined enzyme deficiency. The findings of large numbers of storage macrophages in the marrow of a patient with splenomegaly, hepatomegaly, lymphadenopathy, pancytopenia, cerebral manifestations, malaise, failure to thrive, or other untoward symptoms and signs aid in the confirmation of a hereditary storage disease.

Phagocytic tissue cells that contain in the cytoplasm prominent granules and fibrillar structures that are green, greenish-blue, or dark blue are designated as "**sea-blue histiocytes**." The blue-staining structures are thought to be incompletely degraded pigments and cell membranes. Macrophages with striking blue colors may be a manifestation of a benign condition in which there is a hereditary enzyme deficiency. Usually, the presence of sea-blue histiocytes is an eye-catching nonspecific morphological anomaly.

Phagocytic Histiocytic Malignancies. Malignancies involving mesenchymal cells that are morphologically undifferentiated and those that are potentially or actively phagocytic constitute a large, complex, and overlapping spectrum of diseases which have been given an infinite number of names. Variants which are characterized by the demonstrable ability of some of the cells to phagocytize are monocytic leukemia, histiocytic-monocytic leukemia, and histiocytic medullary reticulosis (malignant reticuloendotheliosis, malignant histiocytosis).

Another entity characterized by cells that have feeble phagocytic properties is "**hairy cell leukemia**" (histiocytic leukemia). Hairy cells have villous cytoplasmic marginal extensions and veillike ruffles. The cytoplasmic protrusions of these aggressive malignant cells tend to push neighboring cells away, leaving wide clear spaces between these cells and adjacent erythrocytes (Plate 42, Fig 23, Fig 25). The nuclei of hairy cells are round or only slightly indented. The chromatin strands are uniformly dispersed, and the nucleoli are indistinct. The cytoplasm stains various shades of blue and reveals a delicate reticular pattern. In some of the cells, there are distinct reddish granules. Some of the cells contain cytoplasmic vacuoles (Plate 42). Opinions differ about the origin of hairy cells. Membrane markers suggest that these cells have features of B lymphocytes. From a morphologic point of view, these cells resemble phagocytic cells rather than lymphocytes. Hairy cells react positively with acid phosphatase stain which is not sensitive to tartaric acid.

Fat Cells

FAT CELLS are seldom seen in thin smears of bone marrow, for they are ruptured in the process of aspiration. When spread on a slide, the contained globules of fat tend to escape and leave the stroma and cell membranes as unidentifiable debris. In thicker portions of the marrow smears, individual fat cells or groups of fat cells can be seen, surrounded by other marrow cells.

Mature fat cells are large round cells, comparable in size to megakaryocytes and osteoclasts (50 to 80 μm in diameter). The small round or oval nuclei are located eccentrically, presumably pushed to one side by the pressure of globules of fat in the cytoplasm. The chromatin structure in many of the nuclei is definite and linear. Often there is a globular body in the nucleus thought to be fatty material in the process of manufacture (Plate 16, Fig 26).

The globules of fat in the cytoplasm are of varying size and are chromophobic or stain a light blue or pink. The fat globules have smooth margins. The globules compress each other, producing irregular shapes. The lipid masses are separated in compartments by cytoplasmic material which appears as delicate blue lines (Plate 16). The fixed character of the cells is revealed by multiple fibrils which extend outward from the cell margins (Plate 16) and interlace with the fibers of fibrocytes and endothelial cells. The lipid material in fat cells has an affinity for various Sudan dyes.

Mesenchymal cells which manufacture fat are to be differentiated from secretory plasma cells with large aggregates of proteinaceous material in their cytoplasm. The secretory droplets in the grape or morula variants of plasma cells are spherical rather than irregular in shape and appear as perfect superimposed circles as if drawn by a small compass (Plate 47). Cells producing fat are also to be differentiated from cells which phagocytize fat, the so-called "lipid-laden" histiocytes or "lipophages." In phagocytic histiocytes, the lipid particles tend to be small, giving to the cytoplasm a foamy or bubbly appearance.

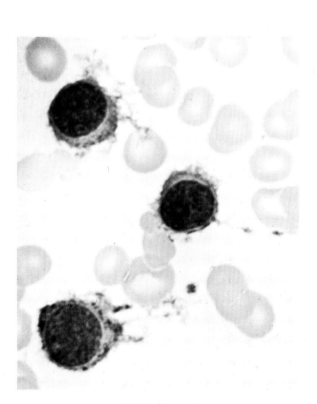

Fig 25 — Hairy cells.

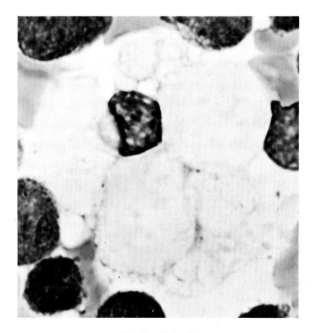

Fig 26 — Fat cell.

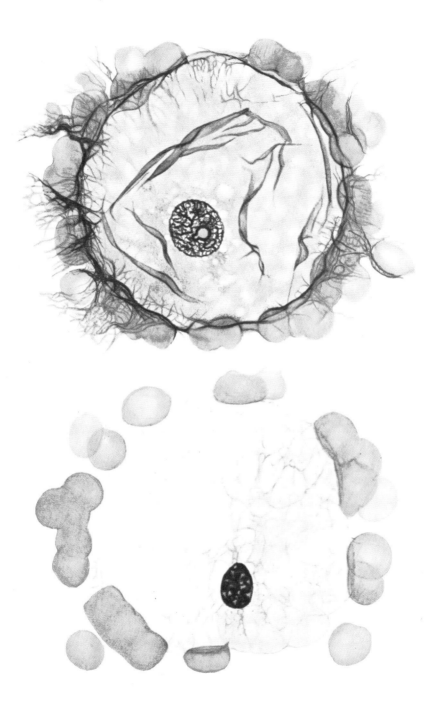

PLATE 16 — FAT CELLS

Top: Fat cell with small round nucleus, linear chromatin and globular body in nucleus, ample cytoplasm with lipoid globules, wrinkled membrane, reticular stroma, and fibrillar marginal structures

Bottom: Fat cell showing cytoplasmic lipoid bodies separated by reticular structures. Structures surrounding fat cells are mature erythrocytes.

Bone Cells

CELLS THAT ARE LOCATED in the Haversian canals of compact bone are designated as "osteocytes." The term "osteoblasts" is used to name cells that are responsible for the formation, calcification, and maintenance of trabeculae and cancellous bone. The destruction and removal of bone is the function of cells identified as "osteoclasts."

Osteoblasts. An osteoblast is a large cell with ample cytoplasm and relatively small, round, and eccentrically placed nucleus (Plate 17). These cells may be traumatized in the process of aspiration and smearing and often have irregular shapes and cytoplasmic streamers. The cells may have comet or tadpole shapes. The nucleus may be partially extruded or may rest outside the cell, like a small round head on a round body. The nuclear chromatin strands and the nuclear margins are well-defined. Usually there is a distinct nucleolus which takes a predominantly blue color in contrast to purple-red stain of the chromosomes.

The basic color of the cytoplasm is blue. Wavy fibrils are often visible. Throughout the cytoplasm, there are small spherical bodies which are colorless and give to the cytoplasm a bubbly appearance. Within the cytoplasm, there is a prominent round or oval zone which takes a lighter stain than the rest of the cytoplasm. This area may be adjacent to the nucleus but is usually away from the nucleus (Plate 17, Fig 27).

Osteoblasts morphologically resemble plasma cells, for both have irregular shapes, pointed cytoplasmic protrusions, blue cytoplasm, eccentric nuclei, spherical bodies within the cytoplasm, chromophobic areas, cytoplasmic fibrils, and vacuoles.

Osteoblasts as a class are larger than plasmocytes. The relatively unstained zone of the plasmocyte is adjacent to the nucleus and partially surrounds the nucleus as a collar, whereas the clear zone of the osteoblast is often distinctly separate from the nuclear margin and when adjacent to the nucleus does not surround or enclose the nucleus. The protein secretions of plasma cells impart a reddish background color which is not demonstrable in osteoblasts.

Osteoblasts in marrow smears often appear in groups or aggregates which may be misinterpreted as malignant cells. The margins of cells in a malignant cluster are indistinct, and one cannot tell where one cell begins and the other ends. Malignant cells are crowded and distorted. The size of the cells and the color and structure of the nuclei tend to be quite variable, whereas in osteoblasts the cells are more orderly and uniform. Light-staining areas in the cytoplasm away from the nucleus are characteristic of osteoblasts and are seldom demonstrable in malignant cells.

CHROMOPHOBIC AREA

AWAY FROM NUCLEUS

NEAR NUCLEUS

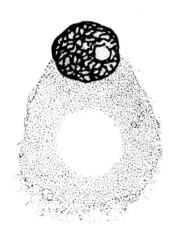

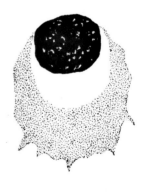

OSTEOBLAST

PLASMOCYTE

Fig 27—Osteoblast vs plasmocyte.

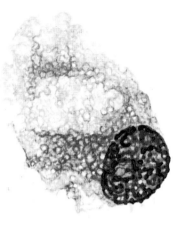

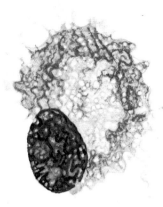

A   B

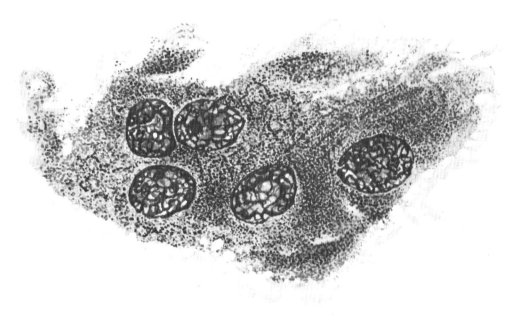

C

PLATE 17—OSTEOBLASTS AND OSTEOCLAST

A Osteoblast with prominent light zone in
   cytoplasm located away from nucleus

B Osteoblast with oval eccentric nucleus,
   distinct linear chromatin and nucleolus, blue
   bubbly cytoplasm with prominent light zone, and
   fibrillar marginal structures

C Osteoclast: Large multinucleated cell with
   uneven number of separated oval nuclei, blue
   granules, and frayed cytoplasmic margins

Osteoclasts. The osteoclast is a very large, irregularly shaped, and elongated cell with multiple round or oval nuclei which are approximately the same size. The number of nuclei is quite variable. The nuclei are separate and are distributed haphazardly within the cytoplasm (Plate 17, Fig 28). It is thought that the large number of separated nuclei within a given cell is due to the fusion of the cytoplasm of multiple osteoblasts into a single large cell (osteoclast). The nuclear chromatin is usually linear, and nucleoli are often visible. The abundant blue cytoplasm has a finely granular or ground-glass appearance. In some cells, there may be distinct granules. In thin smears, it is sometimes possible to demonstrate a ruffled cytoplasmic fringe consisting of diaphanous veils, fingerlike cytoplasmic protrusions, and sacular invaginations.

Osteoclasts and megakaryocytes are sometimes difficult to differentiate, for both may be very large with granular cytoplasm, irregular shapes, and multiple nuclei. The nuclei of megakaryocytes are connected by strands or are superimposed, whereas the nuclei of osteoclasts are usually separated and have no visible connections with each other (Fig 29). The number of nuclei in megakaryocytes is even, whereas the number of nuclei in osteoclasts may be uneven.

Osteoclasts are usually demonstrable in areas where bone is in the process of demineralization and absorption. It is thought that osteoclasts synthesize and secrete enzymes that aid in dissolution of osteoid tissue and calcific bone.

There is evidence that plasmocytes in the bone marrow of patients with multiple myeloma and lymphoid leukemia produce an osteoclast-stimulating factor that helps to explain the development of the osteolytic bone lesions observed in these conditions.

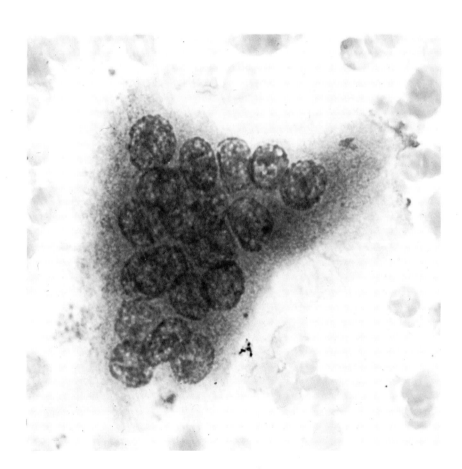

Fig 28—Osteoclast.

Fibrocytes (Fibroblasts)

FIBROCYTES are connective-tissue cells present in blood-forming organs as well as in all other parts of the body. These cells are responsible for the synthesis and secretion of polypeptides (trophocollagen) that aggregate (polymerize, crystallize) into long fibrils. These fibrils form bundles of varying size with varied physical and staining characteristics. They are identified as reticular, collagen, and elastic fibers.

In tissue sections and in cultures, mature fibrocytes are elongated and spindle-shaped cells with oval nuclei, non-granular or finely granular cytoplasms, and multiple branching cytoplasmic protrusions. These cells are not capable of phagocytizing large particles. Fibrocytes are so tightly bound by their intertwined cytoplasmic extensions, by connective-tissue ground substance, and by fibers that they are aspirated with difficulty. They are seldom seen or at least not identified as fibrocytes in smears or imprints of hematopoietic organs.

Although fibroblasts usually are not thought of as blood cells, they are essential constituents of blood-forming organs. After injury to marrow cells due to any cause, there is a proliferation of fibrocytes, producing fibrosis (scar tissue). Malignancies involving fibrous-tissue elements are known as fibrosarcomas. When the malignant process involves fibrocytes as well as other types of bone marrow cells, the condition is known as "leukemic myelosis" (leukemic myelofibrosis, agnogenic myelocytic metaplasia). In Hodgkin's disease, there is a malignant proliferation of lymphocytes as well as fibrocytes and Reed-Sternberg and other cells.

Endothelial Cells

OCCASIONALLY one sees in marrow smears fragments of small intact vascular channels, the lumens of which are bounded by elongated nongranular cells with oval nuclei. Spindle or oval cells may be scraped from the lining of blood vessels or from the heart chambers by the point of a needle in the process of collecting blood. These cells are identified as endothelial cells by their organoid arrangement. Individual endothelial cells are not identifiable.

NUCLEUS

SEPARATED   ATTACHED

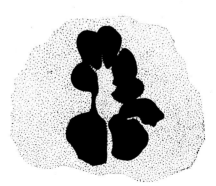

OSTEOCLAST   MEGAKARYOCYTE

Fig 29—Osteoclast vs megakaryocyte.

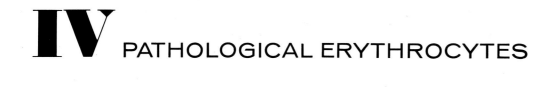

PATHOLOGICAL ERYTHROCYTES

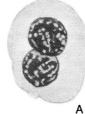

A

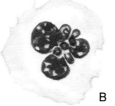

B

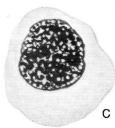

C

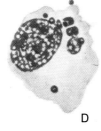

D

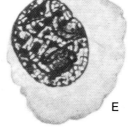

E

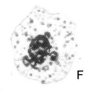

F

G

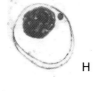

H

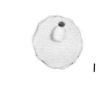

I

J

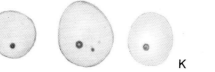

K

L

PLATE 18—PATHOLOGICAL ERYTHROCYTES

A Macrocytic rubricyte with two nuclei
B Stippled macrocytic rubricyte with fragmentation of nucleus (karyorrhexis)
C Macrocytic prorubricyte with asynchronism between nuclear structure and cytoplasmic color
D Macrocytic prorubricyte with nuclear fragments and asynchronism between nucleus and cytoplasm
E Macrocytic prorubricyte with thickening of portions of nuclear chromatin (pyknosis)

F Atypical nucleated red cell with degenerated nucleus and nuclear fragments (? stippling)
G Metarubricyte with partial extrusion of portion of nucleus
H Atypical stippled metarubricyte with Howell-Jolly body and Cabot rings
I Erythrocyte containing malarial ring
J Thrombocyte on erythrocyte
K Howell-Jolly bodies in erythrocytes
L Cabot rings in erythrocytes

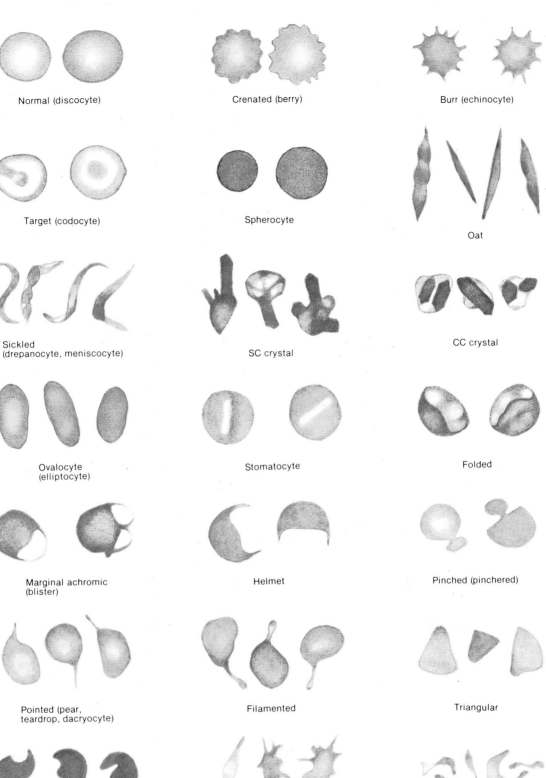

Normal (discocyte)

Crenated (berry)

Burr (echinocyte)

Target (codocyte)

Spherocyte

Oat

Sickled
(drepanocyte, meniscocyte)

SC crystal

CC crystal

Ovalocyte
(elliptocyte)

Stomatocyte

Folded

Marginal achromic
(blister)

Helmet

Pinched (pinchered)

Pointed (pear,
teardrop, dacryocyte)

Filamented

Triangular

Poikilospherocyte
(small, dark, irregular)

Acanthocyte
(thorn, spur, spicule)

Schizocyte
(schistocyte)

Membranous ghost

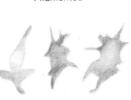

Crescent
(semilunar)

PLATE 19—SHAPES OF RED CELLS

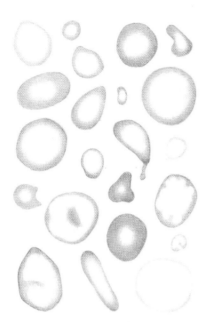

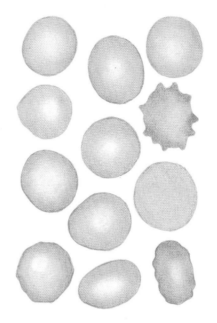

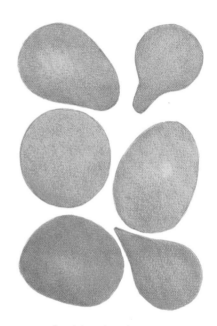

Iron Deficiency Anemia   Normal   Pernicious Anemia

Thalassemia Major   Hereditary Spherocytosis   Ovalocytosis

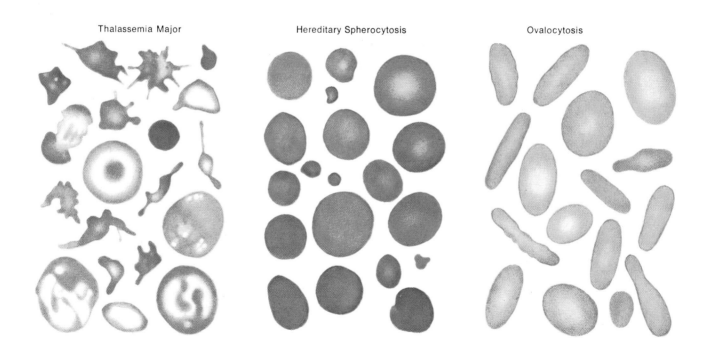

PLATE 20—ERYTHROCYTE MORPHOLOGY IN VARIOUS DISEASES AND SYNDROMES

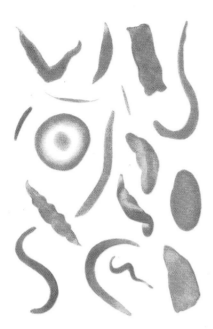

Sickle Cell Anemia

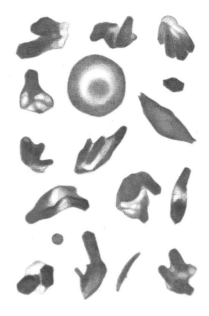

Sickle Cell—Hemoglobin C Disease

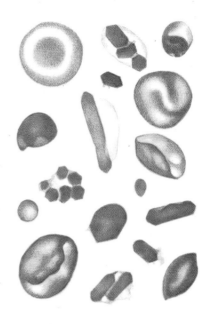

Homozygous C Disease

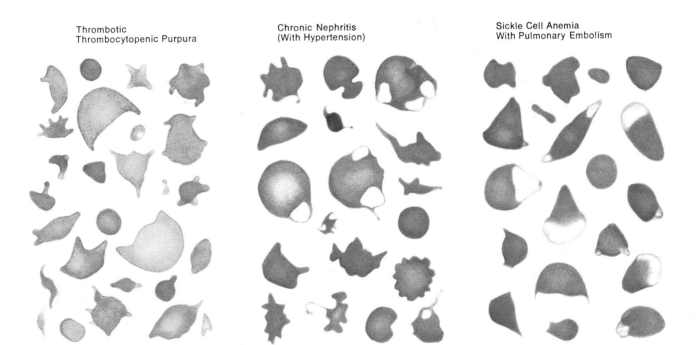

Thrombotic
Thrombocytopenic Purpura

Chronic Nephritis
(With Hypertension)

Sickle Cell Anemia
With Pulmonary Embolism

PLATE 21—ERYTHROCYTE MORPHOLOGY IN VARIOUS DISEASES AND SYNDROMES

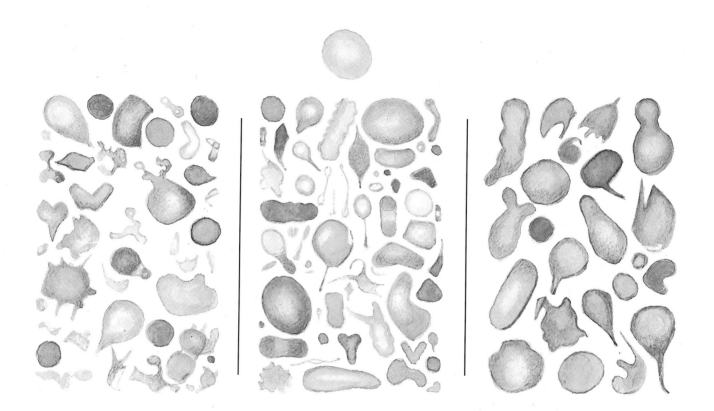

PLATE 22 — SELECTED ERYTHROCYTES FROM PATIENTS WITH BURNS (LEFT),
HEREDITARY PYROPOIKILOCYTOSIS (CENTER), AND MYELOFIBROSIS (RIGHT)

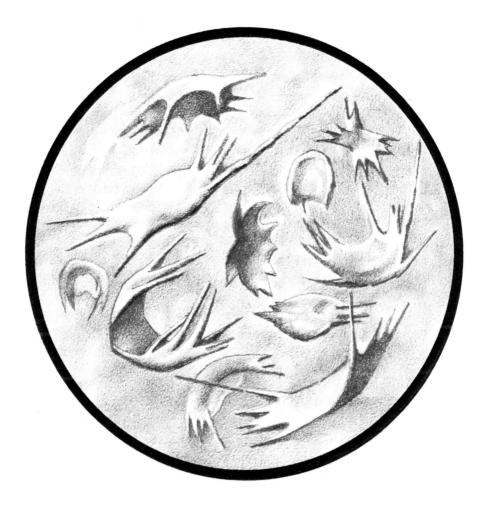

PLATE 23—MOIST UNSTAINED PREPARATION OF BLOOD FROM A PATIENT
WITH SICKLE-CELL TRAIT, SHOWING REVERSIBLE ELONGATED MULTIPOINTED
RED CELLS AND CELLS WITH MARGINAL PROTRUSIONS

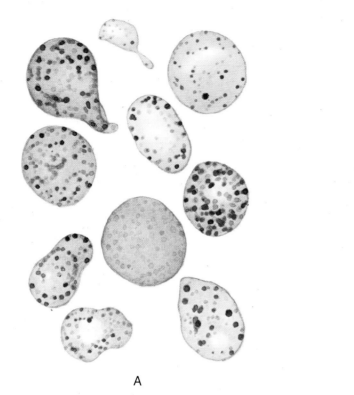

A

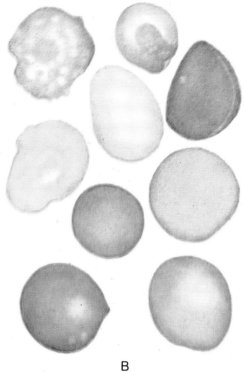

B

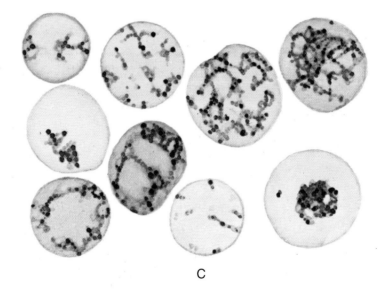

C

PLATE 24—STIPPLED CELLS, DIFFUSELY BASOPHILIC ERYTHROCYTES, AND RETICULOCYTES

A Selected stippled erythrocytes (punctate basophilia) in a Wright-stained blood smear from a patient with lead poisoning.

B Selected diffusely basophilic erythrocytes in a blood smear, Wright stain.

C Selected reticulocytes containing granulofilamentous structures in a smear from blood mixed with new methylene blue stain. Diffusely basophilic cells and stippled red cells are revealed as reticulocytes in a new methylene blue preparation.

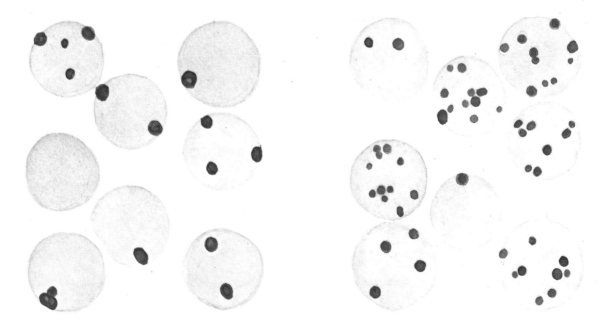

PLATE 25—ERYTHROCYTES WITH HEINZ BODIES

Erythrocytes in a moist preparation after four-hour incubation with acetylphenylhydrazine followed by staining with crystal violet (x 2,500)

Left: Normal blood with one to four Heinz bodies in most erythrocytes.

Right: Erythrocytes from a patient with G-6PD deficiency. Majority of red cells have five or more Heinz bodies.

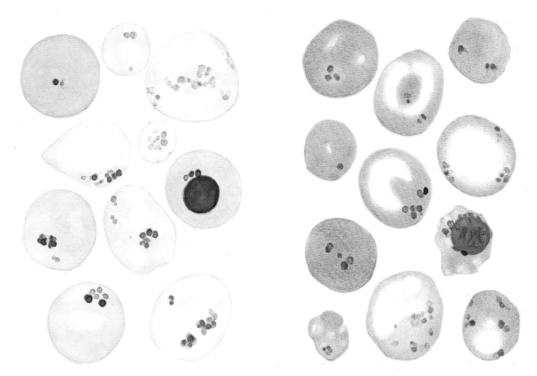

PLATE 26—SIDEROTIC GRANULES IN ERYTHROCYTES

Left: Wright stain showing a metarubricyte and multiple nonnucleated erythrocytes with Pappenheimer bodies (siderotic granules). The granules vary in number, size, shape, and color and are unevenly distributed.

Right: Prussian blue stain for iron showing one nucleated red cell (ringed sideroblast) and multiple nonnucleated erythrocytes containing blue-staining siderotic granules (siderocytes). The nucleus of a nucleated red cell stains red with safranin. (Howell-Jolly bodies, Heinz bodies, and RNA bodies in stippled cells do not give a blue color with the iron stain.) x 2,500

PLATE 27—PERNICIOUS ANEMIA, BONE MARROW

Selected nucleated and nonnucleated red cells in bone
marrow smears of patients with untreated pernicious anemia.
There is asynchronism between nucleus and cytoplasm with
the nucleus less mature than the cytoplasm. Identification of
nucleated cells is based on chromatin configuration and not
on cytoplasmic coloration. Anisocytosis, poikilocytosis, and
anisochromia may be observed in nonnucleated erythrocytes.

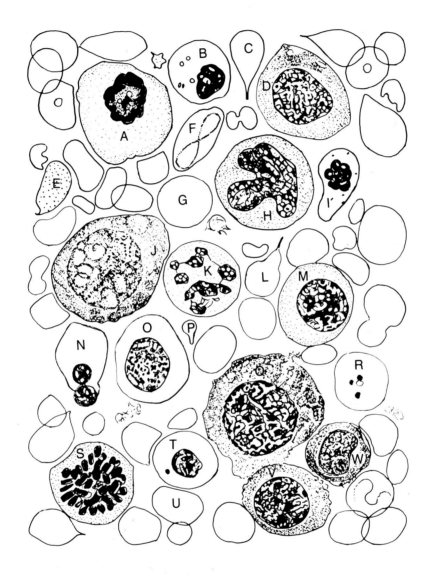

A Macrocytic metarubricyte showing karyorrhexis and
   asynchronism
B Macrocytic rubricyte with Howell-Jolly bodies
C Teardrop erythrocyte
D Macrocytic prorubricyte with immature nucleus and more-
   mature cytoplasm
E Stippled red blood cell
F Cabot ring in oval macrocyte
G Diffusely basophilic cell
H Large lobulated neutrophil
I Metarubricyte showing karyorrhexis and Howell-Jolly
   bodies
J Macrocytic rubriblast (megaloblast) with multiple nucleoli
K Hypersegmented neutrophil

L Pear-shaped erythrocyte
M Macrocytic rubricyte
N Macrocytic metarubricyte with fragmentation and
   beginning nuclear extrusion
O Macrocytic dysplastic nucleated red cell
P Microcytic poikilocyte
Q Macrocytic rubriblast of type observed in pernicious
   anemia
R Macrocyte with Howell-Jolly bodies
S Mitotic figure
T Macrocytic metarubricyte with one Howell-Jolly body
U Oval macrocyte
V Macrocytic prorubricyte
W Prorubricyte

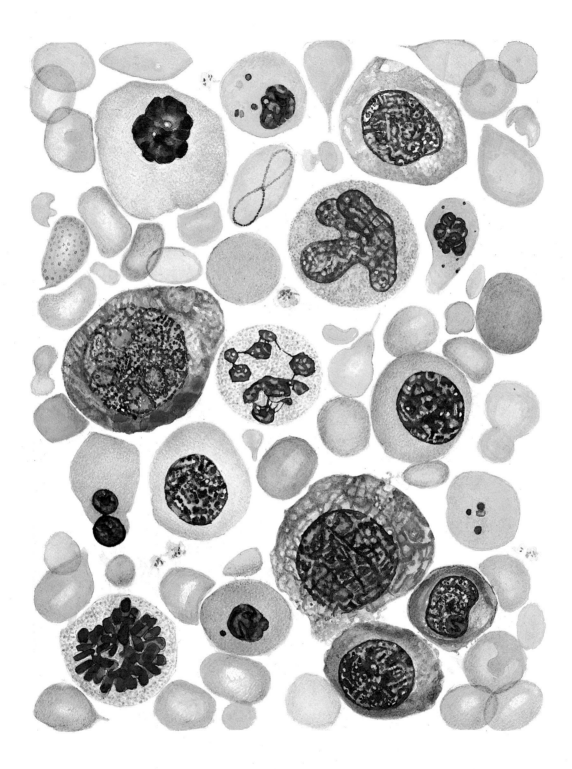

PLATE 27—PERNICIOUS ANEMIA, BONE MARROW

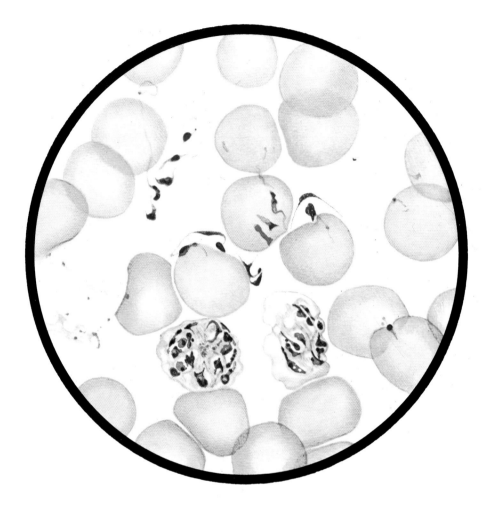

PLATE 28—MALARIAL PARASITES: *PLASMODIUM VIVAX*

Bone marrow, Wright stain. Two malarial schizonts and the stroma
of a ruptured schizont with recently released merozoites.

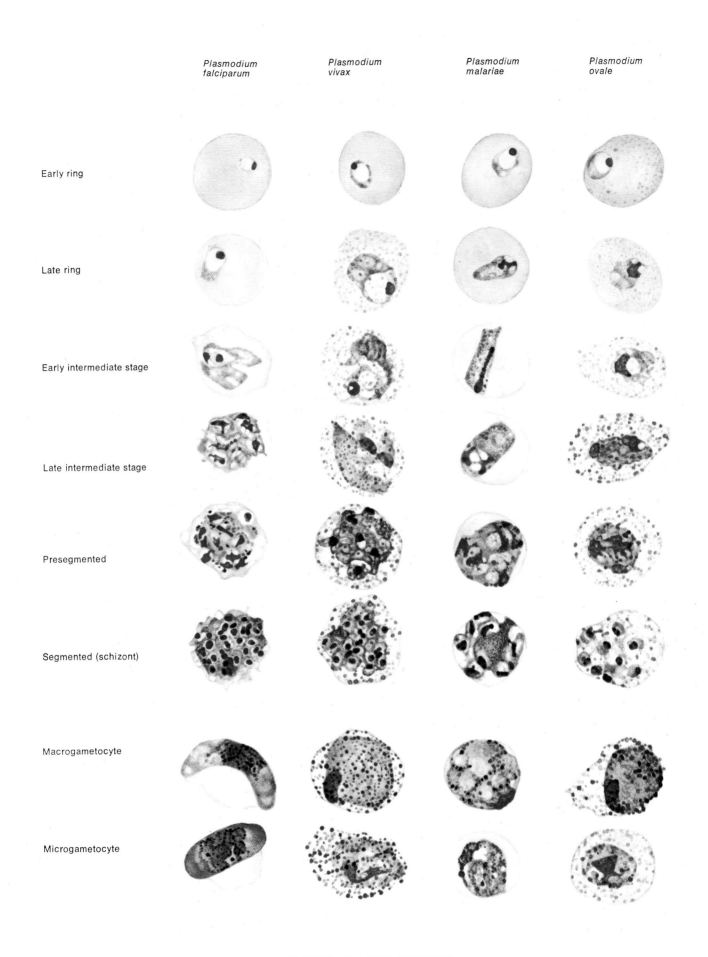

	Plasmodium falciparum	*Plasmodium vivax*	*Plasmodium malariae*	*Plasmodium ovale*
Early ring				
Late ring				
Early intermediate stage				
Late intermediate stage				
Presegmented				
Segmented (schizont)				
Macrogametocyte				
Microgametocyte				

PLATE 29—MALARIAL PARASITES

63

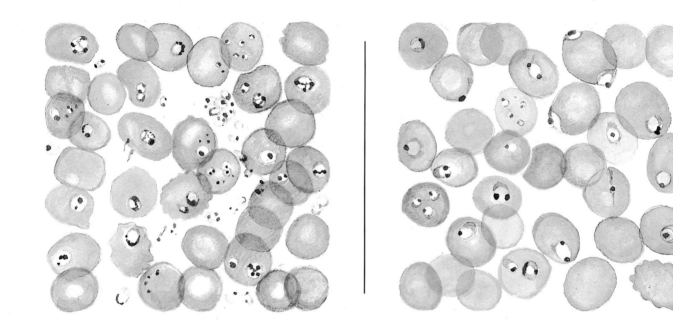

PLATE 30 – PROTOZOAN PARASITES

Left: *Babesia*, intracellular and extracellular parasites
Right: *Plasmodium falciparum*, ring forms

PATHOLOGICAL LEUKOCYTES
AND THROMBOCYTES

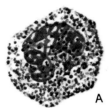

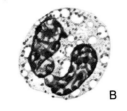

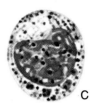

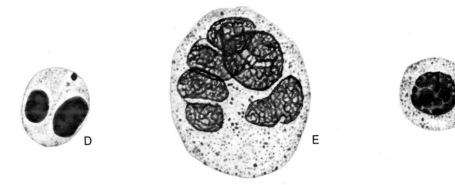

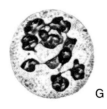

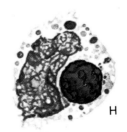

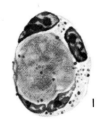

PLATE 31—PATHOLOGICAL LEUKOCYTES

A Neutrophil with prominent dark-bluish granules
(toxic granules)

B Neutrophil segmented with vacuoles, a sign of
degeneration

C Neutrophil metamyelocyte with toxic granules

D Degenerated neutrophil with pyknotic nuclei
and nuclear fragment

E Giant neutrophil with multiple nuclei (polyploid
neutrophil)

F Degenerated (pyknotic) nucleus in a neutrophil
with prominent granules

G Hypersegmented macrocytic neutrophil
(PA poly)

H Monocyte with phagocytized pyknotic nucleus
(Tart cell)

I Segmented neutrophil with purple-staining
cytoplasmic mass from a patient with lupus
erythematosus

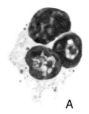

A

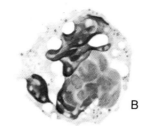

B

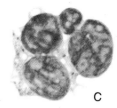

C

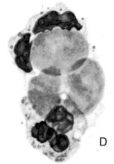

D

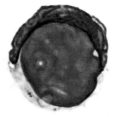

E

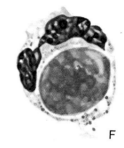

F

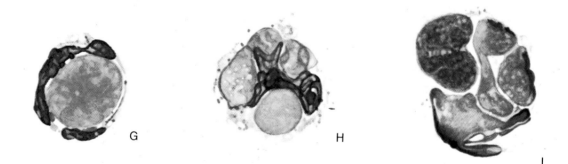

G

H

I

PLATE 32—SO-CALLED "LE CELLS" IN SMEARS FROM PATIENTS WITH LUPUS ERYTHEMATOSUS

A Segmented neutrophil with swelling of lobes and early degenerative changes (pre-LE cell)

B Segmented neutrophil with early lytic changes in nucleus and vacuoles in cytoplasm (pre-LE cell)

C Swelling and degenerative changes in lobes of segmented neutrophil (pre-LE cell)

D Two neutrophilic leukocytes adjacent to lysed nuclear masses. (Large groups of neutrophils around degenerated nuclear material are known as rosettes.)

E, F, G Neutrophils which contain in their digestive vacuoles phagocytized purple or reddish-purple nuclear material from other leukocytes. Cells having this morphology are designated as "LE cells." The structure of the phagocytized mass is not completely smooth and homogeneous but is characterized by light and darker areas with an absence of distinct linear markings.

H, I Degenerative changes in nuclei of phagocytic neutrophils which have engulfed lysed nuclear masses (post-LE cell)

The diagnosis of lupus erythematosus should not be made on the basis of morphology alone but on clinical abnormalities and combined laboratory tests. In deciding whether or not the morphological changes are compatible with the diagnosis of lupus erythematosus, one should appraise the degenerative changes in the cells destined to be phagocytized (pre-LE cells), the degenerative changes in the nuclei of phagocytes (post-LE cells), as well as the neutrophils with phagocytized nuclear masses in their cytoplasm (LE cells).

66

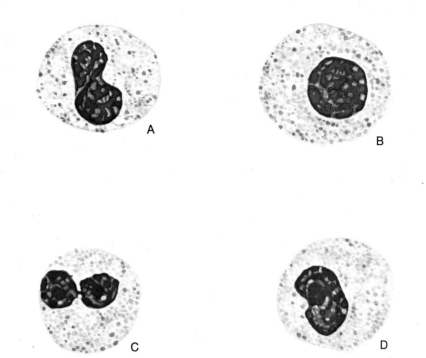

PLATE 33 – PELGER-HUËT ANOMALY

This hereditary anomaly is characterized by hypolobulation of the nuclei of granulocytes. The chromatin structure of the granulocytes with round or indented nucleus is that of mature cells. The size, chromatin structure, and phagocytic function of these cells are normal.

A "Peanut"-shaped nucleus
B Round nucleus

C Nucleus with closely approximated round lobes (pince-nez)
D Slightly indented nucleus

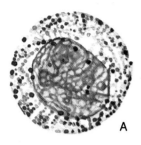

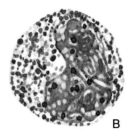

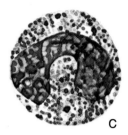

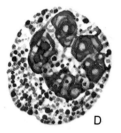

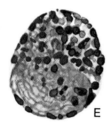

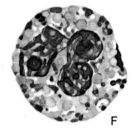

PLATE 34—ALDER'S ANOMALY

A Neutrophilic myelocyte
B Neutrophilic metamyelocyte
C Neutrophilic band

D Neutrophilic segmented
E Basophil
F Eosinophil

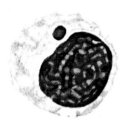

A

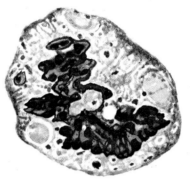

B

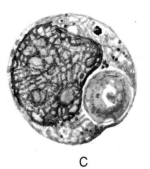

C

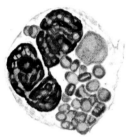

D

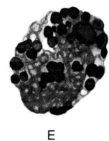

E

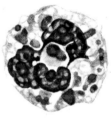

F

PLATE 35—CHÉDIAK-HIGASHI ANOMALY

Leukocytes in smears of peripheral blood or of bone marrow from patients with Chédiak-Higashi anomaly showing abnormal and giant lysosomes in the cytoplasm.

A Lymphocyte
B Promyelocyte in mitosis
C Promyelocyte

D Eosinophil
E Basophil
F Neutrophil

Other variants not shown include giant chromophobic globules, very-dark granules in neutrophils, elongated granules, crystallike bodies, and large anomalous granules in monocytes.

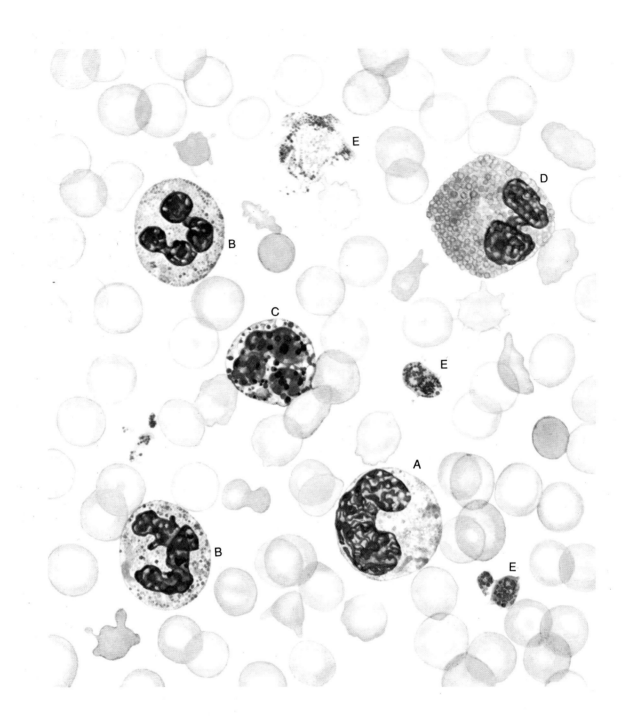

PLATE 36—CELL TYPES FOUND IN A SMEAR FROM A PATIENT WITH MAY-HEGGLIN ANOMALY

A Monocyte with light blue cytoplasmic masses of
  varying sizes and irregular shapes (Döhle bodies)
B Segmented neutrophils with Döhle bodies
C Basophil with Döhle body
D Eosinophil with Döhle body
E Abnormal thrombocytes

*Cells were arbitrarily chosen to show
characteristic abnormalities. The number of
thrombocytes and leukocytes is greater
than occurs in a single oil-immersion field.*

*Note variation in shape of erythrocytes with
crenated, blunt filamented forms and
spherocytes.*

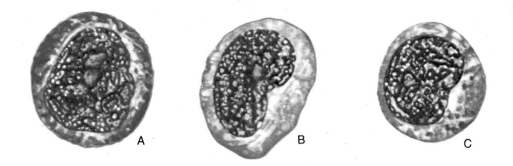

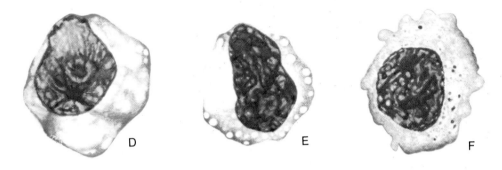

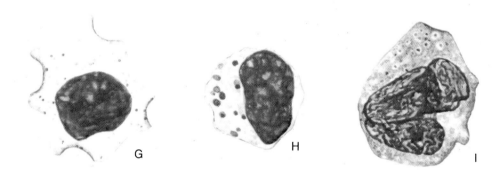

PLATE 37—INFECTIOUS MONONUCLEOSIS

A Primitive plasmalike cell
B, C Plasmalike cells with indented nuclei and
 early nuclear structure
D Large reactive lymphocyte with unevenly
 stained bluish cytoplasm
E Large lymphocyte with vacuoles in cytoplasm

F Atypical monocyte
G Large lymphocyte with azurophilic granules
 and scalloped borders (indented by red cells)
H Large lymphocyte with prominent reddish
 (azurophilic) granules
I Atypical monocyte

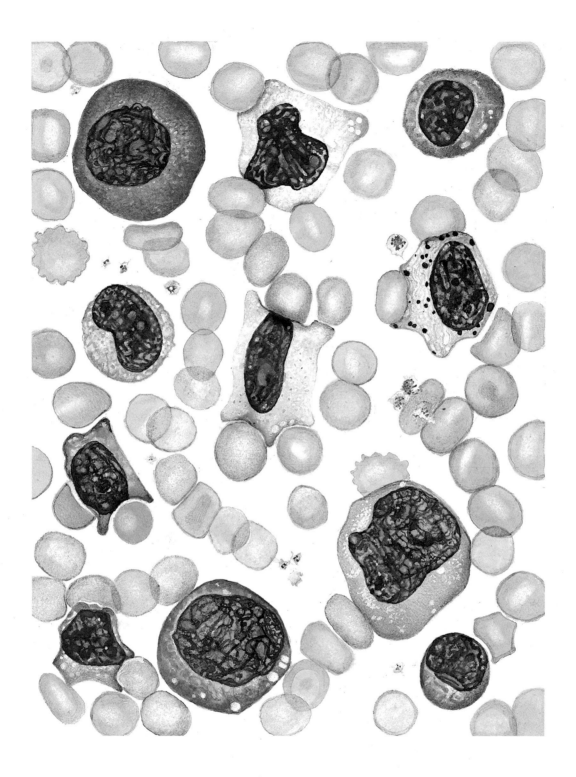

PLATE 38—REACTIVE LYMPHOCYTES

In this color plate the leukocytes other than lymphocytes have been left out. Selected lymphocytes reacting to antigenic stimuli and showing heterogeneous forms have been portrayed in increased numbers in order to reveal the marked variation in size and shape and in nucleus and cytoplasmic characteristics. Note large cells with prominent basophilic cytoplasm, granules in some cells, and indentation of some lymphocytes by red cells. Red cells and thrombocytes are normal.

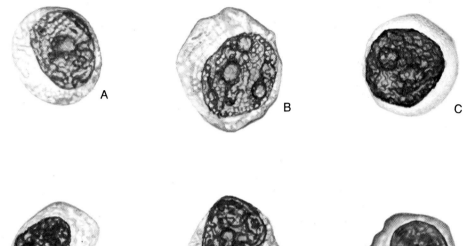
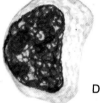
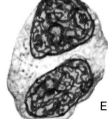
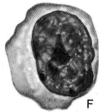
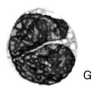
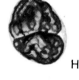

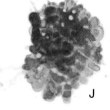

PLATE 39—LYMPHOCYTIC LEUKEMIA

A Lymphoblast with nucleolus
B Lymphoblast with prominent nucleoli
C Prolymphocyte with indistinct nucleolus
(? lymphoblast)
D Prolymphocyte with intermediate chromatin
structure and rippled appearance of cytoplasm
E Prolymphocyte with double nuclei with
immature nuclear chromatin

F Atypical lymphocyte with clumping of nuclear
chromatin, purplish-red nongranular cytoplasm
G Prolymphocyte with deep nuclear cleft
H Lymphocyte with multiple nuclear lobulation
I Lymphocyte with nuclear fragment
J Smudge

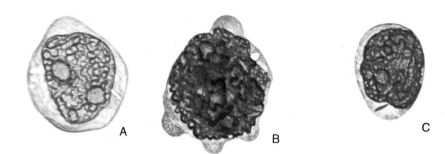

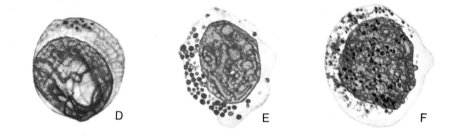

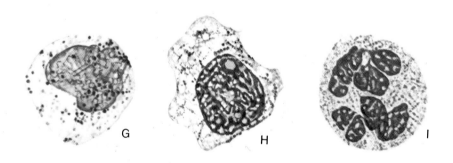

PLATE 40—GRANULOCYTIC LEUKEMIA

A Myeloblast with prominent nucleoli, well-defined chromatin structure, deep-blue cytoplasm, and no granules

B Atypical early cell with dark coarse nuclear chromatin structure and blunt vacuolated pseudopods (probably a micro-megakaryoblast)

C Myeloblast with Auer rod in cytoplasm

D Atypical promyelocyte with occasional dark granules

E Atypical promyelocyte with prominent purple granules

F Atypical promyelocyte with fine and coarse granules

G Atypical large granulocyte (simulating monocyte) with indented nucleus, intermediate nuclear chromatin structure, nonspecific granules, and relatively large amount of cytoplasm

H Atypical immature neutrophil (? neutrophilic tissue cell)

I Macrocytic polyploid neutrophil

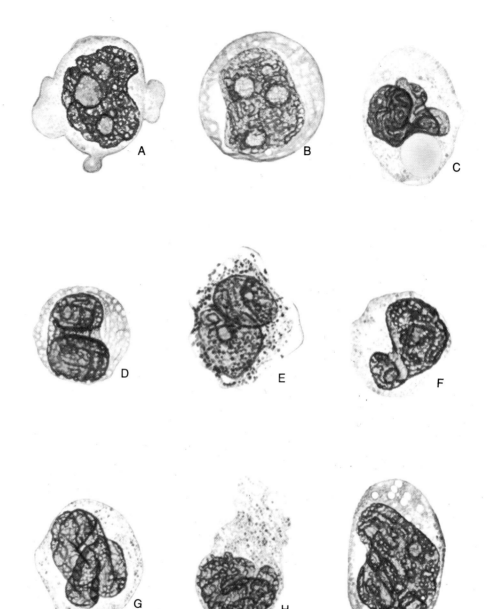

PLATE 41—MONOCYTIC LEUKEMIA

A Monoblast with prominent nucleoli, indented
   nucleus, and blunt pseudopods
B Monoblast with prominent nucleoli
C Monocyte with phagocytized red cell
D Promonocyte with nuclear folds, foamy
   cytoplasm
E Promonocyte with two nuclear lobes, nucleoli,
   prominent granules, and clear ectoplasm

F Monocyte with deeply indented nucleus and
   granular cytoplasm
G Monocyte with transparent folded nucleus,
   granules in cytoplasm
H Monocyte with folded nucleus, linear chromatin,
   distinct granules, and elongated shape
I Promonocyte with nucleoli and vacuoles in
   cytoplasm

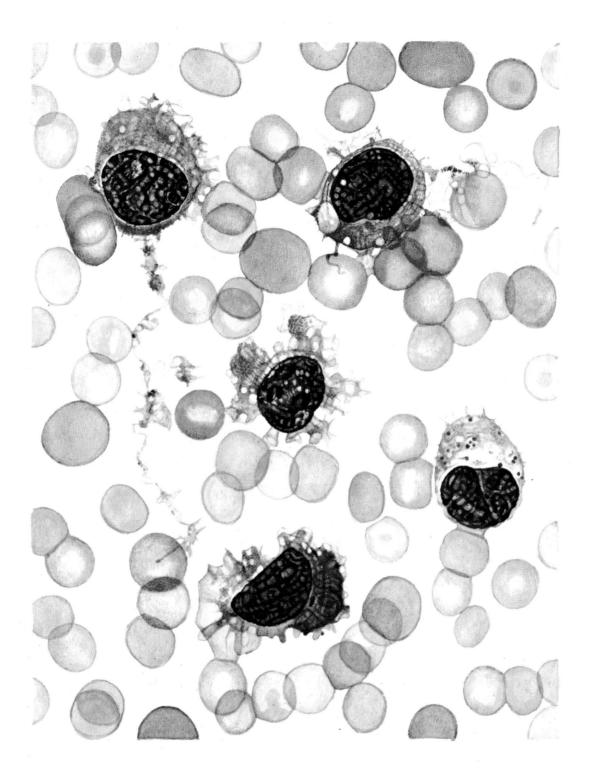

PLATE 42—HAIRY-CELL LEUKEMIA

Selected cells as seen in peripheral blood smears from a patient with hairy-cell leukemia. These cells have veillike cytoplasmic extrusions and delicate threadlike filaments. They tend to push neighboring cells away or aside, leaving clear spaces around the hairy cell.

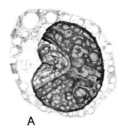

A

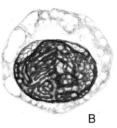

B

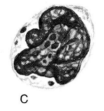

C

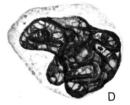

D

PLATE 43—SÉZARY SYNDROME

A Vacuolated atypical immature lymphocyte with
   indented nucleus, fine swirled chromatin pattern,
   and nucleoli

B Vacuolated atypical early lymphocyte with
   distinct chromatin strands

C Atypical lymphocyte of intermediate size with
   brainlike (cerebriform) convolutions and
   granules

D Atypical lymphocyte with nuclear folds and
   blue cytoplasm.

   *Features sometimes seen and not shown
   include nuclear clefts and cytoplasmic
   extensions.*

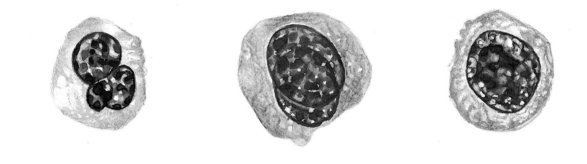
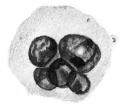
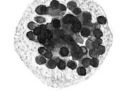

PLATE 44—NUCLEATED RED CELLS IN SMEAR OF PERIPHERAL BLOOD FROM PATIENT WITH
ERYTHROLEUKEMIA (DI GUGLIELMO'S DISEASE)

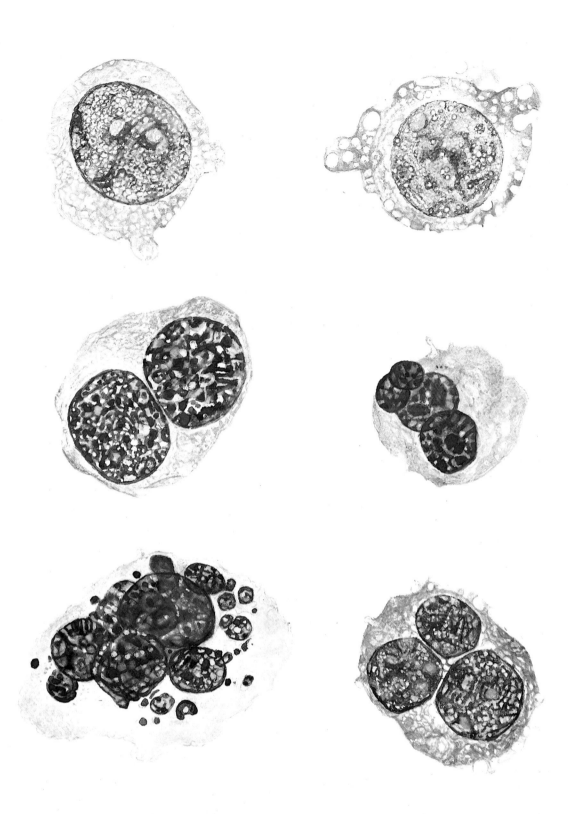

PLATE 45—NUCLEATED RED CELLS IN SMEAR OF BONE MARROW FROM PATIENT WITH
ERYTHROLEUKEMIA (DI GUGLIELMO'S DISEASE)

Note variation in size, vacuolization, multiple nuclei, and nuclear fragmentation.

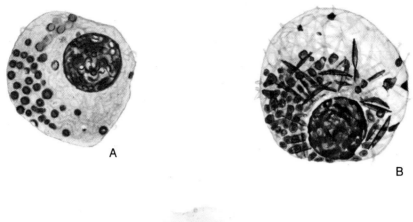

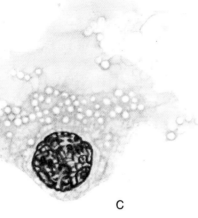

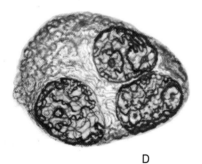

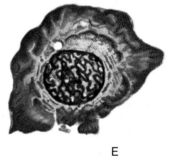

PLATE 46—PATHOLOGICAL PLASMOCYTES

A Plasmocyte with red-staining globules in cytoplasm (Russell bodies) and red-staining material in nucleus

B Plasmocyte with eccentric nucleus and with red-staining crystalline bodies, red globules, and reticulated cytoplasm

C Plasmocyte with nebulous cytoplasmic margin, multiple globules, and pink-staining homogeneous secretory material

D Proplasmocyte with three nuclei and reticular cytoplasm

E Flame type of plasmocyte

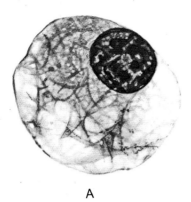

A

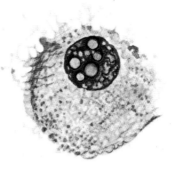

B

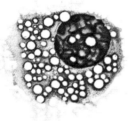

C

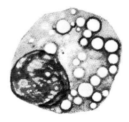

D

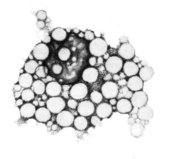

E

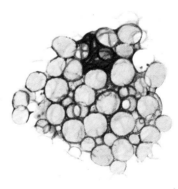

F

PLATE 47—PLASMOCYTE VARIANTS

A   Plasmocyte showing reticular cytoplasmic
    structure
B   Plasmocyte with globular bodies in nucleus,
    reticular cytoplasmic structure, shaggy
    margins, and red secretions

C   Plasmocyte with multiple globules and frayed
    margin
D, E, F   Plasmocytes with globular bodies

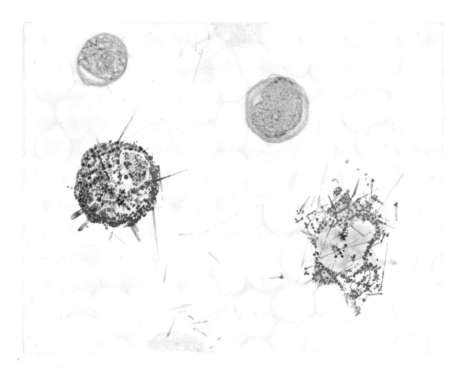

PLATE 48 — PEROXIDASE STAIN (SATO AND SEKIYA)

The two upper cells are peroxidase negative (lymphocytes); the two lower cells are peroxidase positive (granulocytes). The red cells are laked and appear as shadow forms. This stain is of aid in differentiating early cells of the myelocytic and monocytic systems from cells of the lymphocytic system.

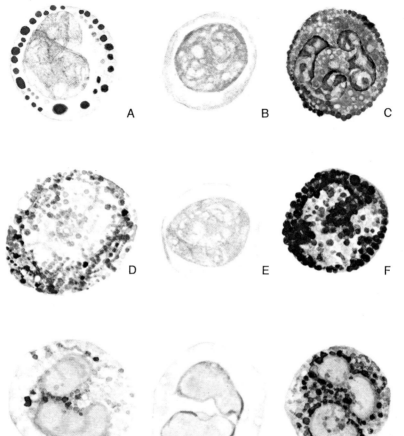

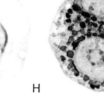

PLATE 49—CYTOCHEMICAL STAINS

Periodic acid-Schiff (PAS) reaction for the detection of intracellular glycogen:

A PAS positive substance in cytoplasm of a lymphocyte from a patient with Sézary syndrome

B Negative PAS reaction

C Strongly positive PAS reaction in a segmented neutrophil

Sudan Black B stain for the detection of lipids:

D Immature granulocyte showing positive reaction

E Lymphocyte showing a negative reaction

F Strongly positive reaction in a neutrophil

Leukocyte alkaline phosphatase stain:

G Faintly positive reaction in a neutrophil

H Negative reaction in a neutrophilic granulocyte

I Strongly positive reaction in a neutrophil

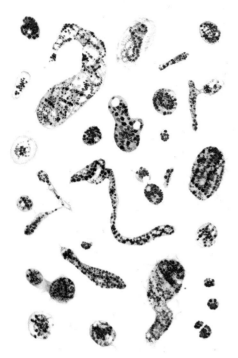

IDIOPATHIC THROMBOCYTOPENIC
PURPURA

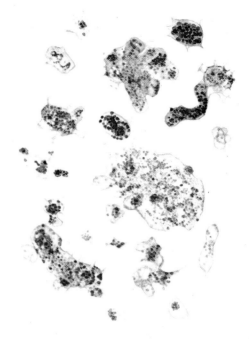

MAY-HEGGLIN ANOMALY

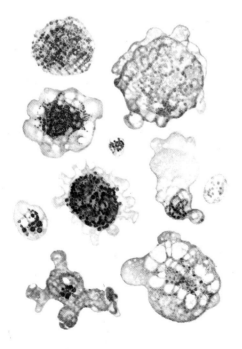

LEUKEMIC MYELOFIBROSIS

THROMBASTHENIA

PLATE 50—PATHOLOGICAL THROMBOCYTES (x 2,000)

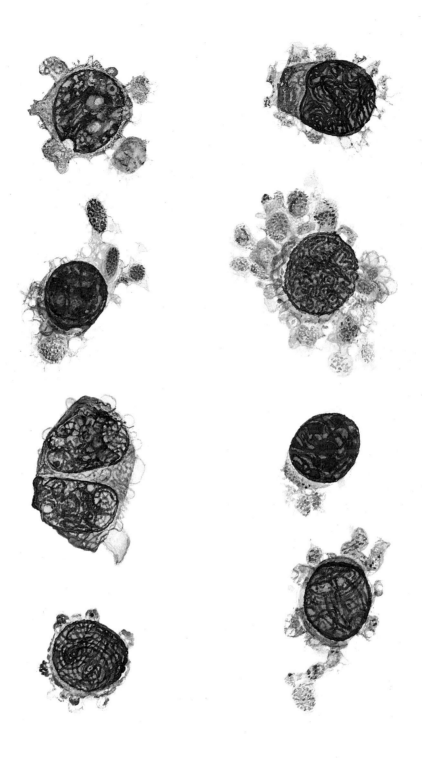

PLATE 51—MICROMEGAKARYOCYTES

Variant forms of small megakaryocytes from a patient with blast crisis of chronic granulocytic leukemia. Nuclei are usually single, but one cell has double nuclei. In some cells, bubbly cytoplasm and variable formation of platelets are noted.

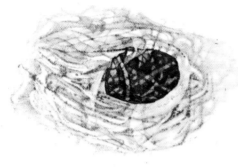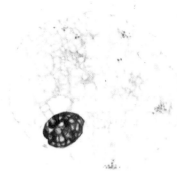

PLATE 52—LIPID HISTIOCYTES

Gaucher's Disease   Niemann-Pick Disease

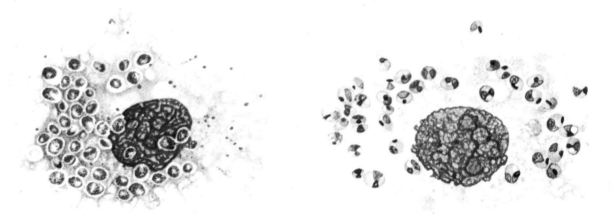

PLATE 53—BLOOD PARASITES

Macrophage with phagocytized   Macrophage with *Leishmania donovani*
Histoplasma capsulatum

PLATE 54

ORIGIN AND DEVELOPMENT
OF
BLOOD CELLS

(on following two pages)

PLATE 54—ORIGIN AND DEVELOPMENT OF BLOOD CELLS

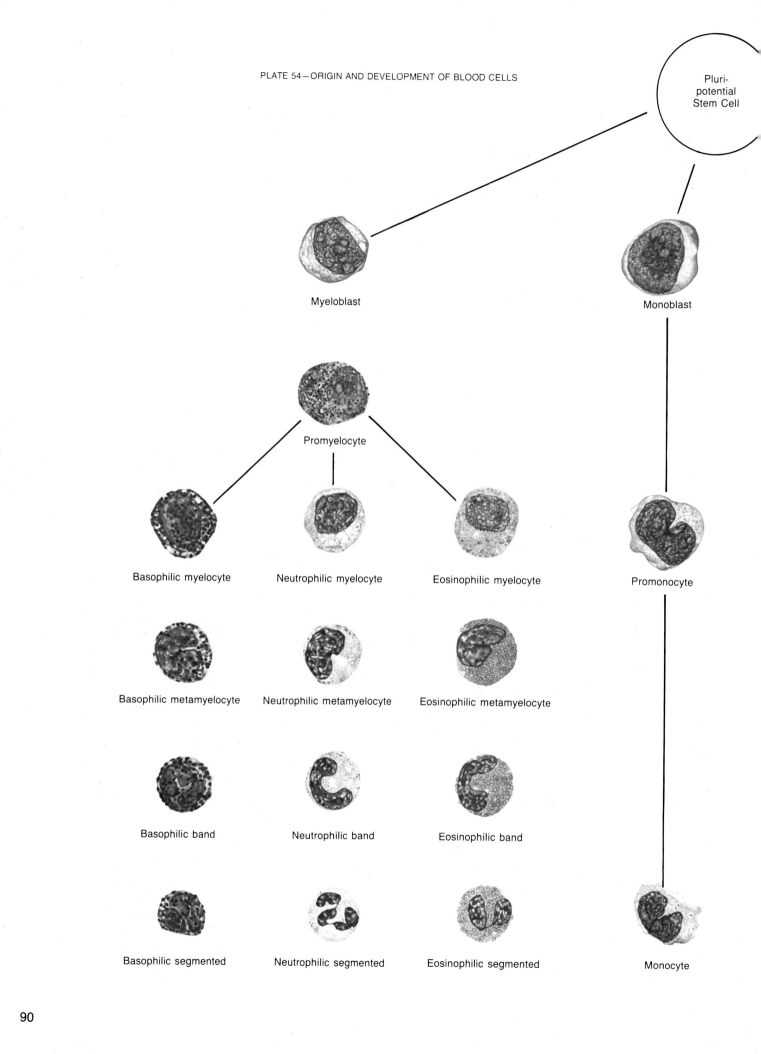

Pluri-
potential
Stem Cell

Myeloblast

Monoblast

Promyelocyte

Basophilic myelocyte

Neutrophilic myelocyte

Eosinophilic myelocyte

Promonocyte

Basophilic metamyelocyte

Neutrophilic metamyelocyte

Eosinophilic metamyelocyte

Basophilic band

Neutrophilic band

Eosinophilic band

Basophilic segmented

Neutrophilic segmented

Eosinophilic segmented

Monocyte

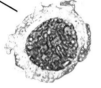

Megakaryoblast

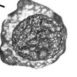

Rubriblast

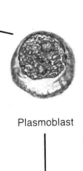

Lymphoblast

Plasmoblast

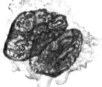

Promegakaryocyte

Prorubricyte

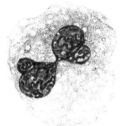

Megakaryocyte
without thrombocytes

Rubricyte

Prolymphocyte

Proplasmocyte

Metarubricyte

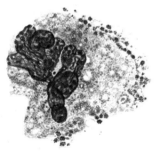

Metamegakaryocyte

Diffusely basophilic
erythrocyte

Thrombocytes

Erythrocyte

Lymphocyte

Plasmocyte